Gastric Sleeve: The New Me

Project preview

M Mitchell

Published by FastPencil Publishing

Table of Contents

My name is Mindy Mitchell. I had the sleeve gastrectomy (also known as gastric sleeve) on November 3, 2015. I'm thirty-three, married, and have four children. I'm writing this book in hopes of sharing my journey with others as my life changes daily and moves forward. Moving toward the good. Progress is a daily walk and not a run or a race to the finish line. Many times you will go on diet after diet after diet but still end up only losing water weight. I have tried everything from low carb to paid various companies for shakes, supplements, and certain food. All were a failure for me because before you can change your eating habits, you have to change your mentality and eating habits. Some people have underlying conditions that prevent them from being successful at dieting, which was my case. Weight loss is a life changing experience that takes months even years.

Many people will say "Wow Mindy! What diet have you been on because you look great!" I give them the honest truth. I tell them I had the gastric sleeve. The next questions people ask are about what diets have I tried, why did I take such a drastic measure, and did I do it to look better? My decision wasn't based on any type of physical appearance. My surgery decision was about saving my life. If I had not had the surgery, I probably would not be here to tell you about my journey. I chose my surgery because it was my last option after surviving a stroke at thirty-one, seizures, narcolepsy, and issues with high blood pressure. When you have a stroke at thirty-one, you wake up and realize its time to do something drastic. Sometimes you have to do something drastic to save your life. Regardless of what others think, they will criticize you for your decision, but, ultimately, the decision is yours. If you let others make your decisions for you, you will never outgrow the person you are used to being. This is referred to as living your life to please others. I mean, come on, get real with yourself. If you are constantly doing what others tell you, you become a toy for them to control. By taking control of your own self, you take control of your future.

The Sleeve Gastrectomy may not be your choice as far as weight loss surgery, but it was mine. There are other surgeries out there including the Lap Band and Gastric Bypass. I personally did not choose the Lap Band due to the requirements every month of coming in to tighten and loosen it up. I also wanted a permanent fix. I personally did not choose the Gastric Bypass because I wasn't interested in the after effects of the surgery related to my intestines and rerouting my insides. The Gastric Sleeve was my best option because it was a permanent fix and less invasive. I am happy with my decision. The time leading up to my surgery and the road that this journey has taken me on before and after surgery has changed me as a person. I have become a better person to myself and to others. Throughout my book, I'm going to share my journey from my ultimate decision to the person I have become after my surgery. I hope you get something out of my journey to help you along yours. Sleeve brothers and sisters for life!

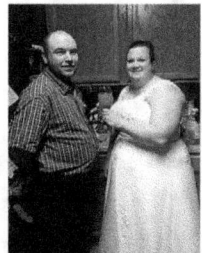

Our One Year Wedding Anniversary

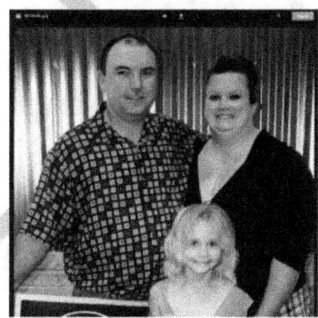

Picture of Me and My Husband the Summer Before My Surgery (at 189 lbs)

The Struggle Is Real

The Struggle Is Real

The struggle is real. Deciding if you really are hungry or if it's your mind playing tricks on you. Even after surgery, my mind plays tricks on me. The issues that brought me to the plate aren't available in my life anymore. It's just my brain signaling to my mind that it's noon and the time on the clock says it's time to eat, but my stomach says no. Passing by the refrigerator or the kitchen doesn't affect me like it used to.

The struggle is real when you see fast food signs and think of the old you wanting and craving that burger and fries you saw on the road sign. When you see it, you want it. When you get it and taste it, it doesn't taste as good as it used to. Tastes are different after surgery. The foods I used to enjoy make me sick now. The smell of grease makes me sick.

The struggle is real and it is a struggle daily to keep pushing forward. I have found things to do during the time I used to spend searching for food during times of boredom. The struggle is hit head on when you finally realize this is the struggle you will have for the rest of your life.

My Past Health History

There's so much to write here that I have absolutely no idea where to start, so I guess I'll start at the beginning. This is the beginning of my journey and how I ended up where I am now. It has definitely been a long journey, but glad to be where I am and happy for where God is taking me throughout my journey. Your destination starts with a beginning. Here is mine.

Up until I was twenty three, I weighed one hundred twenty five pounds. I have always been lean and thin my whole life. I never gained a pound. I could eat anything and everything I wanted without any worries of gaining any weight from my food choices. I can remember being a young child and eating one whole pack of hot dogs at one sitting. I never gained an ounce or a pound. I would fill up on hot dogs, Ramen noodles, chips, candy, and everything my heart desired. I always maintained my weight well and had no medical issues either.

When I was in college, I got pregnant with my daughter, who is eight now. I got pregnant with her in 2006. Up until then, like I said, no worries and could eat whatever I wanted. At some point in my pregnancy, I got it in my head I was eating for two and would definitely eat for two thinking to myself "Oh yeah, I'm just gaining baby weight". Little did I know, I was gaining 'body mass weight' as I call it. I went from one hundred twenty five pounds to two hundred twenty five within those nine months. I had also gained a "friend" called gestational diabetes.

During the first three to four months of pregnancy, I gained over forty pounds. I had no idea why I was gaining weight so fast during these first few months, but after a routine visit to the doctor, I figured out why. You would think being thin my whole life that this wouldn't be an issue for someone of my thin frame. Gestational diabetes can hit anybody. I also relate a lot of weight gain to a lot of sleeping from my body changing to a gestational diabetes state.

What I thought was pregnancy tiredness was really my body turning into diabetic. I had to prick my finger three times a day during my pregnancy and was on a special diet throughout it. My body was undergoing a lot of changes and my metabolism was slowing down. At my heaviest during pregnancy, I topped out at two hundred sixty five. I had gained well over one hundred pounds during my pregnancy. This weight gain also showed when I gave birth to my daughter weighing in at eight pounds and nine ounces. She was a butterball. During the first six months postpartum, I lost weight all the way down to two hundred thirty five. I was never able to go back to the weight I had been at my whole life. My body had undergone so many changes throughout pregnancy that it was a struggle to regain my metabolism back and get my body back to its original size pre-pregnancy. Gestational diabetes ended after giving birth.

During this postpartum time, I worked out, went to the gym, and took care of my daughter as a single mom. I even tried different diets without any success. From the time she was born, up until post gastric sleeve surgery, I constantly gained weight over the next seven years up until now. When my daughter was a toddler, it was easy to fix something little for her like a pizza or noodles or finger foods and then eat what she was eating to keep from preparing two meals, one for me and one for her. This can lead you also to failure when dieting. Kids have a higher metabolism than us adults and can burn off calories and weight faster. As adults, we require higher quality foods high in lean protein and low in carbs. Toddler and children's foods contain a lot of carbohydrates. They are made to taste good to young children, but deadly for weight gain for adults. If I could go back and change my eating habits then, I probably would have been a lot healthier during the past seven years, instead of constantly gaining more weight. Oh the things we wish we could change!

The past seven years of her life, I wasn't able to participate much in her activities because I was out of breath and underlying medical conditions presented themselves. When I was twenty six, I was diagnosed with narcolepsy. My weight at this time was two hundred forty pounds. I had gained five pounds during the first years of her life. I had always had a suspicion of something being wrong. I had wondered since all of this weight gain why I was so sleepy all the time and why I had a hard time getting up. I was also falling asleep at work. I used to spend my one hour break taking a nap at work in the break room just so I could finish my shift for the day. At night, I would wake up and have insomnia. Many times, I thought I needed a CPAP machine to help me sleep better. I ended up doing a sleep study after getting a referral to a wonderful doctor I still see today. After two sleep studies, I was diagnosed with narcolepsy and put on amphetamine medication to stimulate me in the morning time. I also took Ambien at night to sleep. The amphetamines made me over stimulated at work and I would run on my feet all day taking care of Alzheimer's patients only to come home and crash out from exhaustion. There is a huge difference between narcolepsy and exhaustion. I can remember falling asleep in public places, such as my car, church, and sitting at a red light just a split second. The amphetamine salts did their job and kept me awake during the day to function properly. I ended up losing some weight. I lost weight down to two hundred twenty. Narcolepsy is a medical condition that must be treated with medications. It can cause you to fall asleep in public places or even behind the wheel. It can cause you to lose focus of daily tasks, as well as cause you to go to sleep and sleep excessively. Exhaustion is not a medical condition, but a temporary condition of the body when it has run out of energy. I was at two hundred twenty at the age of twenty six. I was still overweight and my Body Mass Index (BMI) was in the Obese category. Although I was taking my medications as prescribed, I was still just maintaining the same weight, give or take ten pounds. I was on my feet eight hours a day at work and did more exercise than one can imagine doing at the gym. Still maintaining and not losing weight. I look back at this time and realize now that this was just water weight fluctuating.

At twenty-eight, I was no longer working in the nursing field, but was starting out in the insurance business. I became a licensed agent and started selling auto, home, life, and property-casualty insurance. At this time, I started having issues with going numb, falling out, slurred speech, and dizziness. I was diagnosed that year with Petit Mal Seizures. My seizures were directly related to weight gain and health issues. I weighed in at two hundred sixty five at this time. Being in the insurance business, you do a lot of eating out and fast food because you are constantly on the road travelling or going to business meetings. At business meetings, there were always easy grab foods, like chips, cokes, cookies, and donuts. I don't recall ever being at any of these meetings and seeing healthy foods. By this time, I had pretty well given up on trying to lose weight. I had come to the conclusion that I was never going back to my thin frame. I spent many days and nights shopping and not being able to find clothes that fit anymore. When I did buy a new outfit, it was from the "big girl plus size" store. I had longed to be able to go back to shopping in junior and regular sizes. I can remember walking the mall in huge baggy clothes and flip flops because the only pants I could find to fit were stretch pants and pants with an elastic seam. I wore flip flops because I could not find any tennis shoes that were comfortable. I was wearing a twenty four in pants/jeans and a 3X in shirts along with a size eleven in shoes. I wasn't big, I was just overweight terribly. Throughout my insurance selling days, which lasted about three years, I would eat out with my colleagues as much as possible, ordering whatever I wanted off of the menu, disregarding the calorie intake and other "deadly" things that contribute to weight gain, such as carbohydrates. There are some carbohydrates that are good for you and some that are not. I just happen to be misinformed and truly had no competent knowledge on how to truly be successful at dieting.

What we sometimes think we are doing right, we are really doing wrong. All you ever hear on TV is "Try this diet. Try that diet". Well honey, not to be mean, but those are diets that only a few will be successful at. To be successful at dieting and losing weight, you have to understand and know what your own body is doing with what foods you put into it. Dieting isn't a one size fits all where one thing works for everybody. Then, you have this thing called a "Crazy Wrap" that you wear for eight hours a day and it helps you lose weight. I mean get real with yourself. This is just a temporary fix even if it does work for a while. If you give in to these instant fixes and fad diets, you are selling yourself short. These things aren't a way to maintain your overall health and weight.

At 29, I met my husband Brandon. We met online through his sister-in-law who happened to be my long time friend for years. He has been the greatest man to ever be by my side. He loved me at my heaviest and still loves me at my thinnest. I was two hundred seventy when I met him. He has never made a mention of my weight since we ever met. He always told me I was beautiful and weight didn't matter. At 29, my daughter was five years old. I can remember not being able to get up on her bed and read to her at night because I was so heavy the bed would sink in. I couldn't jump on the trampoline with her nor could I pick her up without hurting myself in some form or fashion. I thank God every day for Brandon. He has been there to help coach her soccer team and other sports because I was too big to do it. At thirty-one, I married Brandon. I was at two hundred seventy five pounds. I can remember shopping for a wedding dress and when I was looking on the racks, all of them were too small for my size. I can remember going into the dressing room to try them on and they were too tight to zip up in the back even when I tried to suck my gut in. My arms were flabby and fat sagged down on the sides. I can remember having to buy a DD bra just to lift my breasts up enough to find my stomach. I had other issues related to being overweight that prevented me from taking care of myself like I should be able to. Brandon had to help me shave, clip my toenails, paint my toenails, get up and down the stairs at our house, carry in groceries because my heart would beat so fast I would have to sit down. He helped me carry clothes baskets up and down stairs. I couldn't stand more than an hour on my feet due to a condition called Plantar Fasciitis. I had so much weight on my body that the Plantar Fasciitis had taken over my feet. I would get up in the middle of the night and need help to go to the bathroom because with all of my weight, I couldn't stand up on my own. Our bed had a permanent indention on my side where I slept. The weight of my body made this indention. I would have to go to physical therapy to try and recover the use of my feet because of the heel pain from Plantar Fasciitis. If only those doctors and therapists could see me now. I laugh at myself at this thought. Their solution was always try different exercises or have the Plantar Fasciitis surgery. The real solution was to lose a lot of weight.

This was the year I also went on high blood pressure medications. I went for what I thought were panic attacks in April of 2014. It wasn't panic attacks at all. It was high blood pressure. My blood pressure was so high in the doctor's office that many times they would make me stay until it would go down to normal ranges. My BMI at this point was 43%. I was in the morbidly obese category. I was going to the gym daily for an hour and running my heart out on the treadmill. Looking back, my body was really too heavy to be running the treadmill because my body wasn't in a position to be exercising. There are so many people who run to the gym first to get in shape without recognizing that the gym is definitely needed, but not a requirement to lose weight. Before you start a workout regime, you should always contact a professional to help create a customized fitness plan specialized for your body. Many people are in the gym doing more damage to their bodies than doing exercise to better their body. I used to think I was out to burn calories. There are few people out here that should be constantly running the treadmill. Losing weight at the gym has to come from a combination of getting your blood pressure up as well as toning exercises. Going to the gym ultimately aided in my body experiencing a stroke.

Two months later, on June 21, 2014, I suffered my first stroke at thirty-one. If you think it can't happen to you, you are wrong. A stroke can happen to anyone at any age. I can recall it like it was yesterday because my stroke was my decision and turning point in my life. My stroke was my wake up call from God that it was time I did something about this weight and help myself. If you won't do it for yourself, at least do it for your children and family. A stroke can take you out at anytime. I am just lucky that I recovered from mine very well with very few complications. Sometimes, God will use ashes from a tragedy in your life to be your stepping stone to something beautiful. This is what happened to me that day right in front of my daughter.

All day on June 21, 2014, I had been feeling terrible and felt like I was having seizures all day. I really wasn't having seizures. I was having early signs of a stroke, but didn't know it at the time. I, like everyone else, blew it off thinking it's just something else. June 21, 2014 was my wake up day and turning point. My husband had went two doors down to a neighbor's house to mow her yard that evening. I was in my recliner I am known for sitting in right in front of our front door. I could see my daughter and her friends outside playing and riding bikes. I was watching TV in my chair. I felt my right side go numb and my first thought was a "charlie horse" or a seizure coming on. I grabbed my blanket and pulled it onto my legs because I was cold and felt chilly as well. My daughter came in the house about an hour after I started feeling this way. I remember telling her to "Go get daddy because I needed help". He never came because she told him to come home when he was done. Apparently, she misunderstood me. He ended up coming home two hours later to find me slumped over in my chair. He managed to get me in the car and drove me to the emergency room. I ended up sitting in the emergency room for five hours until he had to go and get a medical physician to put me in a room of my own because I was experiencing auras. I don't remember much about that night except experiencing auras and the numbness in my side. At some point, I got admitted and woke up the next morning on an IV and head gear on my head testing my neurological system. I ended up spending five days in the stroke unit for evaluation. My legs were so swollen I could barely get out of bed. I was sick at my stomach and my whole body was weak. The neurologist determined I had a stroke from my blood pressure being so high.

It registered at 170/105. I was at stroke levels and had to take blood thinners and more medications over the next year. I also had to take physical therapy to gain strength back in my arms and legs. Although many others have experienced worse effects from a stroke, I consider myself to be very lucky to have escaped with only a few issues including short term memory loss. My blood pressure causing my stroke was directly connected to carrying around so much weight. Since experiencing my stroke, I have gone through a lot health wise up until after my gastric sleeve surgery.

Having a stroke was my turning point, as it became a mission afterwards to get my health back. I consider my light stroke as my wake up call to take better care of myself. My family depends on me and without me, they will fall apart. Having a stroke put a lot of things into perspective for me. I realized then, that without going and seeking help, I was destined for an early death. When your weight is so high that you don't see your own weight on the BMI scale at your doctors office, then it's time to do something about it. I can remember trying to sort it out in my head and justify my weight by making excuses for myself. The only excuse I had was none. There was no excuse for my actions and behaviors that led up to me gaining more weight. After doing some research online, I came across the gastric sleeve surgery.

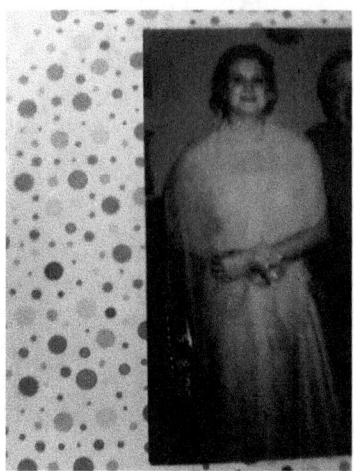

This was me growing up

Taking that First Step

Taking the first step to weight loss is making the decision that it's time for a change. Time to iget up and get moving. Time to figure out what you need to do to get to where you are going. The fastest route may not be the easiest route. Choose the best route for you and your body. Nobody knows your body but you. After researching my different options, from the gym to the surgery, I finally decided on the surgery. Surgery is such a drastic option. Death is not an option for me. If I didn't do anything to change my health, I was going to die. Death from obesity just wasn't in my vocabulary. I had too much to live for. Searching for a surgeon to perform your surgery shouldn't be done by just looking in the phone book. Word of mouth from others, as well as asking your own Primary Care Physician for information, will help you a lot.

After researching the different types of surgeries that were available to me, I made my first appointment about the matter with my PCP. After an hour discussing the pros and cons of what I was considering, we mutually decided that I would be a great candidate for weight loss surgery. Her biggest concerns were my overall health and recovery from the surgery. She had actually had the surgery too. I discussed with her the surgeons I had researched as well. I got referrals to each of them. There were the only three I had to choose from. I went to each appointment I had been referred to. The first surgeon did not think I would even survive the surgery due to having been the victim of a stroke. His influence and advice just made me want to fight harder to seek the advice from another physician. The second surgeon was in Guntersville, AL. He thought I would be an excellent candidate for gastric sleeve and that since it was less invasive that I would have success with it. The third surgeon was in Huntsville, AL close to the first surgeon I had went to see for advice. He did not think I would survive after the surgery because I was borderline diabetic and had high blood pressure. I'm sure you know who I chose. Yes. The surgeon in Guntersville, AL, even though he was over an hour ride from where I lived. I really respected him because he had great bedside manners and pretty well told me what to expect. He was truly a blessing to have. He had my health as his top priority. He asked many questions. He went over how the surgery works and what effects after the surgery I would have. I have always thought great things of him. In the end, he was right and held up to his word. I have been successful beyond more than I can ever imagine. He has taken care of me throughout the entire process and afterwards.

After meeting with him to discuss the options for my gastric sleeve surgery. He gave me a list of requirements for my insurance to be able to pay 100% of my surgery. No doubt I was scared and worried about putting in all the work required just to have insurance later shoot me down. I also learned I had to do nine months of a supervised weight loss diet, as well as complete other medically required appointments just to be able to get insurance to pay. Insurance is always a nightmare and will ask you to jump through a lot of hoops just to get the surgery paid for. It may seem like a lot, but it is well worth it. I assume they drag you through this just so you know how major of a surgery you are about to have. If you don't commit to get your list of things done, you ultimately won't get your surgery. I figured they are just making sure who they invest their money in is going to succeed. I used this time as a teaching moment for myself. I learned as much as I can to help myself in the future. Your decision to have the surgery ultimately depends on your commitment to the insurance company to get them to pay for it. The surgery for me was well over $50,000.00. I had a $0 copay and the only thing I paid was for my required mental health evaluation that was $150.00 out of pocket.

Taking that first step out and taking a leap of faith may seem hard to do, but in the end it is worth it. If you want to do something about your health, you have to first DO something. Taking your commitment seriously will be the reason you actually do succeed. If you decide to change, don't just talk about it, do it. In the end, you are the one paying the consequences for your decision whether you do the surgery or not. My advice for you is to do your research, visit as many doctors as you can for advice, and make your own decision. Don't let others make the decision for you.

The fear of the unknown will keep you from discovering what you should know. If you fear taking the first step, reach inside yourself and figure out what exactly you are trying to accomplish. Without an end in mind, the beginning will never begin. As much as I was scared of the surgery and the idea of my life being at risk, I knew I had no choice and there would be no turning back. If you are constantly looking in the rear view mirror, you will miss what lies ahead. Fear can either lead you away from doing something or it can lead you to doing something great. The feeling of fear is in reality the fear of worry and doubt. Worry and doubt will force you to always think of the negativity in any decision. When I started my journey, I decided then and there that I would only think of the positives in the decisions I was considering. When you fill your head with positive thoughts, positive actions and feelings will follow. I couldn't control what would may happen to me before, during, and after surgery or how others saw my personal decision to get my life back, but the one thing I could and still can control is my own thought processes and my attitude. Your attitude determines your altitude. If you think something bad is going to happen, then it will. Getting the right mindset before you start your weight loss journey will carry you through to the finish line. This is your journey, not anyone else's. I encourage you to stay positive and get in a positive mindset before you make the biggest decision of your life.

Figuring Out The Pay

The wildest beginning of my weight loss journey was dealing with the insurance company. When we hear the word "insurance" our hearts sink to the floor and all we can think about is co pays and how much money we have to pay. Insurance companies are really set up to profit off of you staying sick. For the money they spent on my surgery ($50,000) they could have easily paid for all of the requests I had asked for years ago. I spent years requesting a dietitian, weight loss diet physician, and a medically supervised diet. All of those were denied. The insurance company could at least pay for a portion of the gym membership. At least do something to help people lose weight. Instead, they would rather leave people in obese and sick status and bank on them not figuring out there are other options. More money is spent on weight loss surgery than spent on helping their patients get healthy. It's a terrible truth, but just the way it is. For my own health insurance, they requested a whole page of requirements to be completed before they would allow my weight loss surgeon to apply for my surgery to be performed and paid for by the insurance company.

My individual list started with 9 months of a medically supervised diet by my PCP which included weigh ins, dieting instructions, better food choices, and checks on blood pressure. I was also required to have a colonoscopy, upper endoscopy, mental health evaluation, clearance from a cardiologist, clearance from a lung specialist, clearance from my PCP, physical therapy clearance, and seeing my surgeon a few times up until my information was submitted for insurance to pay. The hardest thing during that time was the waiting game.

While waiting to move on to the next step with my insurance, I missed a lot of work. I spent a lot of during this time waiting for closure from them so I could move forward. The scariest appointment was the upper endoscopy because I was so sick afterwards. They do the upper endoscopy to look for polyps in your stomach. You have to have a stomach free of polyps before you can have the surgery.

The mental health evaluation is really done to discuss the food choices that led you up to being overweight and what changes you are already implementing. They are really just looking to see if you have any underlying conditions such as anorexia or bulimia. The appointment lasts about an hour and also includes drawing a picture of your future plate of food. I know. I felt so stupid and ridiculous. I felt like I was being criticized the whole time. This appointment was a breeze for me, but was mostly irritating. I don't know how anyone can determine if you have an underlying eating disorder by sitting with you for an hour. One good thing came out of this appointment. I learned I was an emotional and boredom eater. I would go to eating when I was bored and eat when I got stressed out. The psychiatrist really encouraged me to take up a hobby to do when I feel the need to eat out of boredom or eat from emotional problems. I have since taken up writing. Writing has become my outlet to express my feelings and thoughts. It has become my way of therapy. Writing helps me to work through the things eating food used to soothe. When you take your focus off of the negative habits and focus on positive habits, you will eventually lose the bad habits. My therapy while working through my doctors appointments was working. I read books and worked extra hours at my job to keep my mind focused and on track for my surgery.

To be approved for surgery, you must clear a cardiologist. A cardiologist clearance consists of getting on a treadmill and determining if your heart rate gets too high or stays within normal ranges. They truly just want to make sure you can maintain your blood pressure during exercise after surgery. This was the appointment I hated the most. Being thin my whole life, I wasn't accustomed to the treadmill or going to the gym. I can remember having to talk myself through my appointment to keep from quitting. No doubt I was ready to get off the treadmill and go home to rest. I was exhausted from being on the treadmill for so long. Five minutes seemed like an eternity to me. I did my best to keep my positive attitude and my mind right. I tried not to think of the pain in my legs and feet, but what kept me going on the treadmill at the doctor's office was my ultimate desire and drive to save my life.

Just when I thought I was done with my pre-surgery requirements, I found out I had to see a pulmonologist. I had no clue what a pulmonologist was, but figured it out soon enough. She turned out to be a doctor checking my lungs. When I was in college, I was on asthma treatments, which made it easier to understand what was going on with me. The pulmonologist was the quickest appointment I had during my pre-surgery time frame. The pulmonologist (lung doctor) is checking for the effectiveness of your lungs while exercising. They are just making sure your lungs are healthy enough to maintain breathing while exercising after your weight loss surgery. Your lungs play a vital role in your blood pressure and heart functions. Some people like myself used to suffer from COPD. COPD causes breathing issues when you try to exercise. The test at the pulmonologist just consisted of breathing treatments and testing how your lungs were functioning before and after breathing tests.

Many of my appointments were back to back. During the six to nine months of pre-surgery requirements, I saw one or two doctors each month getting medical clearances. The insurance company required me to undergo a physical therapy evaluation. A Physical therapy evaluation is a usual required test by the insurance company. They ask for a physical therapy evaluation so they will know you are able to exercise after surgery. The physical therapist goes through a routine of tests that involve bending and stooping and lifting weights. They are looking also to determine what weights your body can handle. This gives the doctor a starting point to figure out how to help you achieve your weight loss goals easier without a lot of stress on your body. Having Plantar Fasciitis made this really hard on me because I spent my doctors appointment hoping and praying I would be able to stand up on my feet without the heel pains. I had the best physical therapy team. They sent me home with tools and ideas to use at home to help my Plantar Fasciitis. They showed me exercises I could do at home as well as after surgery to help ease the pain in my heels. I did pass. They also gave me great recommendations after my surgery.

After all of these appointments, you get to the point where you are just exhausted and feel like you have been checked out on all ends. This may seem like total turmoil seeing different doctors every day but it is truly in your best interest. Your surgeon is trying to make sure your body can withstand surgery. My surgeon was great at staying on top of things for me and was there for me at each stage of the process of going through the insurance requirements.

The insurance circle will lead you into circles. Expect lots of calling back and forth to the doctors and the insurance company. Insurance is a circle in itself. Once you think you have completed all of your requirements, you have to go back to one of your evaluations and get the doctor to reword the documentation correctly so you can get an approval. After getting through the nine months of my insurance requirements, it was time to get prepped for my surgery. It was a long exhausting process, but also a great learning process for me. I learned how to better take care of myself as well as what to expect after my surgery.

Eat for Surgery

The pre-op diet is the scariest words you will hear throughout this process. A small set of words formed to make a sentence that will make your stomach turn in knots. When I first heard them, I felt the same way. I felt a lot of nervousness, strength, and confusion, not knowing what to expect, much less if I could actually follow through with it. My determination led to my own commitment to doing everything I needed to do to succeed. When you finally come to the point of commitment, you change your mindset. In life, you learn that the only one you can commit to in bettering yourself and your life is you. Nobody is going to better you but you. Having will and determination will take you further in bettering yourself than spending time wondering what others are going to think. Lots of people in your life will look at you like you are crazy when you are on your two week or three week pre-op diet. My particular one was two weeks. I can remember waiting for my pre op appointment and I was so excited because I had gotten the go ahead from my insurance company. All I could think about was how hard I have worked during the 6+ months I spent fulfilling the requirements for my insurance company just to approve my surgery.

The thought of the pre-op diet for me never truly hit home until I got into the appointment the Thursday before surgery and listening to my nutritionist tell me everything I needed to know to have me ready for surgery a week later. The first thing she gave me was a small serving cup. It was barely bigger than a shot glass. It fit in the palm of my hand. The first words out of her mouth were: "After surgery, this cup is the size of your stomach. Your stomach will be this size and will only hold half a cup of food". I'm like WOW. Literally, I had no words because I was in such shock. My first thoughts were "how am I going to live on half a cup of food?" I guess where there is a will there is a way. Most of the appointment dragged on about how my diet and eating lifestyle would be changing to include more proteins. I was too fascinated by the idea of my stomach only holding half a cup of food. The half cup was broken into three sections. The first half of the half cup was to be filled with proteins, whether it be beans or a similar protein. Then, on top of the half cup, was 1/2 vegetable, and the last portion 1/2 carbohydrate to total the whole 1/2 cup. It was then I realized how much of a lifestyle change I was fixing to undergo.

After the explanation of the size of my stomach, she gave me a folder. Inside was a list of the foods I would never eat again. The list was longer that I expected and each food item on it made me sad at how much I wish I had known before I gained all this weight. Basically, all processed foods were on the list. No chicken nuggets, canned foods, fried foods, fries, burgers, hot dogs, and all other foods not fresh and greasy. All of the foods I am used to eating were basically put on the NO list from now on. It was this day I learned WHY and HOW I ended up at my heaviest weight. This was also one of my turning point days. One of the days you decide you aren't going back. So, I'm sure you are wondering what I could eat on the pre-op diet. Honestly, it wasn't much. By the time you cut out half the grocery store, there's not much left but fruits and vegetables from the fresh section of the store. The nutritionist gave me a strict diet to follow. I won't lie. It was hard to not want to run to McDonald's drive thru and get fries and burgers and things you are used to eating. I found myself at times struggling between my mind and my stomach craving things I shouldn't be eating.

The first week, up until 72 hours before surgery, the nutritionist put me on a strict diet of fresh fruits and vegetables. I had to count all of my calories to stay under my 1800 calorie mark. I had to eat things like hummus, jello, and high protein vegetables. I can remember spending my last week before surgery buying Steamfresh protein blend bags from the frozen foods section of the grocery store and bringing them home to individually bag into portion sized snack bags. I prepared them and kept them in my freezer for grab and go at work as well as on the run. I would pack myself a lunch daily of carrots, apples, applesauce, and hummus bags to dip my carrots in. I carried two to three bottles of water with me and sometimes brought a banana. For breakfast, I was required to drink Slim Fast shakes. They weren't too bad as long you drink them ice cold. All of this dieting was to shrink my liver in preparation for my upcoming surgery.

Shrinking my liver was the goal by the time surgery date came. This was a daily struggle for me. When you pass drive thru restaurants, you have the urge to stop and buy something you enjoy eating. I would find myself feeling like I was dying of hunger and sit in the car outside burger king and cry my eyes from my taste buds seeking that burning desire for a cheeseburger. I had to put myself on a schedule all day to keep myself from eating so that I didn't spend all day munching on junk food. The struggle was real. Lots of times, I would tell myself that just a few bites won't hurt but in reality, if you aren't eating what you are supposed to eat, the surgery won't happen. I won't lie. I did cheat a little on the pre op diet.

The struggle between your mind and your taste buds will drive you over the edge sometimes. Being able to control your hunger is a lesson you will eventually learn throughout this process. The pre-op diet will give you a test of your commitment to changing. During my pre op diet time, I learned many lessons. The main one being that I AM IN CONTROL of my eating. As humans, we sometimes lose control of our eating when we lose control of our emotions. My family thought I was crazy during my pre op diet because I was so obsessed with making sure that I completed my requirements that I got my mind set that nobody was going to stop me. When others want to put you down and tell you you can't do and shouldn't do it, ignore them and stay focused. You are in control of you. It's time to take care of you.

Don't let anyone tell you their opinion or laugh because you are eating jello and sugar free puddings and hummus. This surgery is about you and without the pre op diet being followed to shrink your liver, things aren't going to change for you. The pre op diet will help you with your eating afterwards. By the time you have completed it and had surgery, you will already have found foods you enjoy eating and like. This isn't a race but a jog to the finish line of getting your life back.

I can remember bringing home my packet from the nutritionist thinking this was something I would never be able to accomplish. I read my diet shopping list many times over and over again. I even took it with me to the grocery store to keep me on track. You will drink lots of fluids and learn to drink water, not in moderation, but all day every day. The pre op diet will help you with your fluid intake as well. After surgery, your success will depend on your fluid intake. The pre op diet will teach you about what you can and cannot snack on to stay on track with your diet. Your pre op diet prepares you for two things: before surgery and after surgery. Don't give up and if you make a mistake, get right back on track!

You will eventually find new foods you like and after surgery, the foods you used to eat don't taste the same. During my pre op diet, my taste buds changed. When I removed sugar, bread, carbs, and processed foods from my diet, I began to crave more veggies and proteins. Your body will signal you and tell you what you need. You just just have to learn to read the signals. I even started to feel better while I was on my pre op diet. I lost 18 pounds on my pre op diet during those two weeks preparing for surgery. My blood pressure went down to normal ranges and I wasn't so sluggish. I was thirsty a lot and did my best to stay hydrated. The pre op diet will either make you or break you. It will force you to do the impossible, which is succeed. I cheated a few times on my pre op diet, but I didn't let it stop me from getting right back on track.

Many of my friends who have had the surgery worry about cheating for a meal. They worried themselves into thinking they weren't going to get to have the surgery because they cheated on their diet. Truth of the matter is, even if you do cheat once or twice, you can still have the surgery. The idea is to shrink your liver, but truly why would you want to gorge yourself with more food knowing that after surgery, you will have more weight to lose on top of the weight you already have to lose. I encourage everyone considering weight loss surgery to have one last meal of food you enjoy eating because after your surgery, it won't even taste good to you. My bucket list of foods I savored for the last time were wonton rolls, crab rangoon, pizza, fried chicken tenders, Captain D's fish, and fries. There will be a day you can eat these again, but you will eat very small portions. You aren't eliminating these foods forever. You will just eat them in moderation. My husband, daughter, family, and friends helped me to have what I called a "food funeral".

A "food funeral" is a meal where you savor everything you truly enjoy eating from your past life before you prepare for surgery. You invite people who love you and care about you over to your house or favorite place to eat. You prepare or buy all the foods you are going to miss and have a buffet of food you will be saying goodbye to. A "food funeral" was great for me because it helped me to see and realize how much greasy and fatty food I was actually eating. My "food funeral" put my old diet of eating anything and everything into perspective.

A "food funeral" helped to bring closure to my past eating habits as well. Looking back, I laugh about the occasion because at the time I felt like I was hugging a friend goodbye that I know I'll never see again. It was a bittersweet moment and a moment of true empowerment on my behalf. It helped me to gain control of my thoughts and opinions of food and the way I looked at food. My view of food had been skewed for so long. My comfort wasn't going to depend on food anymore because deep down I know I had worked so hard to get to this point in my journey. Why destroy something I had worked so hard to achieve? Achieving my goal of saving my life was in the palm of my hand. The pre op diet was just a stop along the way to getting towards the end of my journey. When I had come this far and made it to my pre op diet, I knew there was no time to waste and no more wasting time to destroy all I have worked for during the preparation process for my surgery. Saying goodbye to the "old" and hello to the "new" is like giving birth to a new beginning. My new beginning started when I made my choice to turn my life around. God has given me that opportunity. I would not have made it through a stroke and epilepsy without Him providing me with His perfect timing and love. The timing He provided for me for my surgery came after I had spent much of my younger adult life going through the struggles to teach me how to rise up against the enemy. The wrong foods were the devil and the enemy to me. Fueling up on fast food and processed foods were slowly killing me and allowing the devil to take over my body. The pre op diet became one of my saving grace moments. I hope you are blessed with many saving grace moments during this part of your journey too.

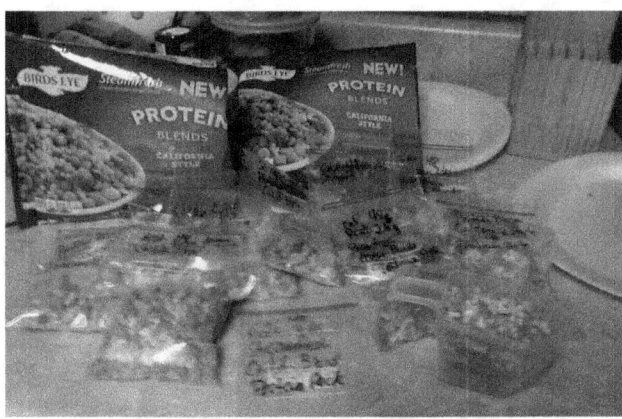

Things You Will Have to Do

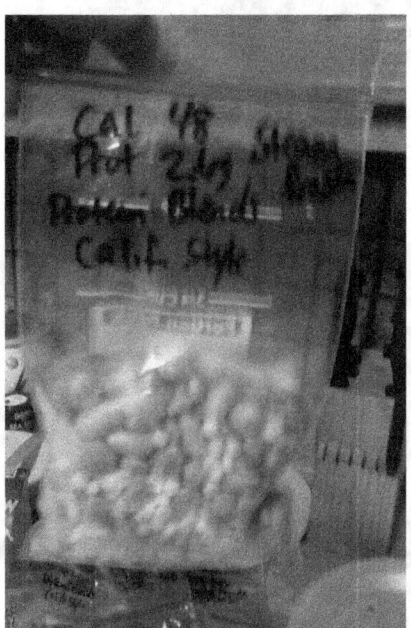

Pre Op Food

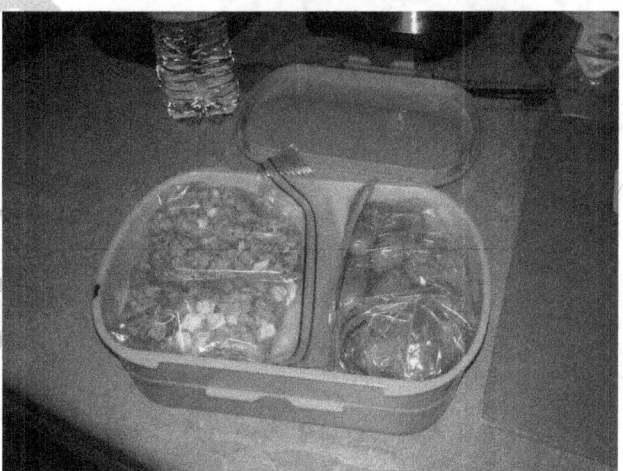

Sample of my Pre Op Lunch

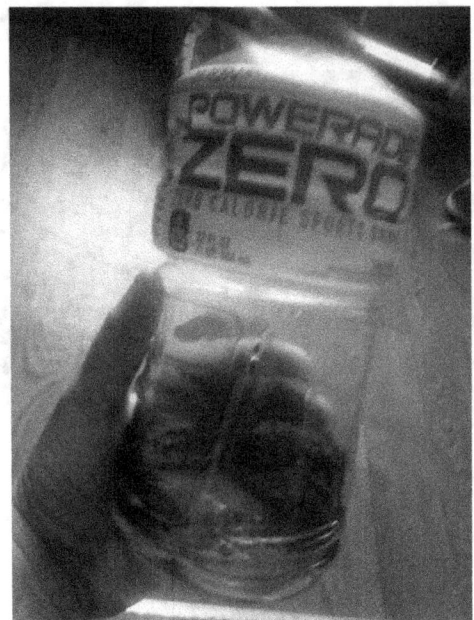

Clear Liquids

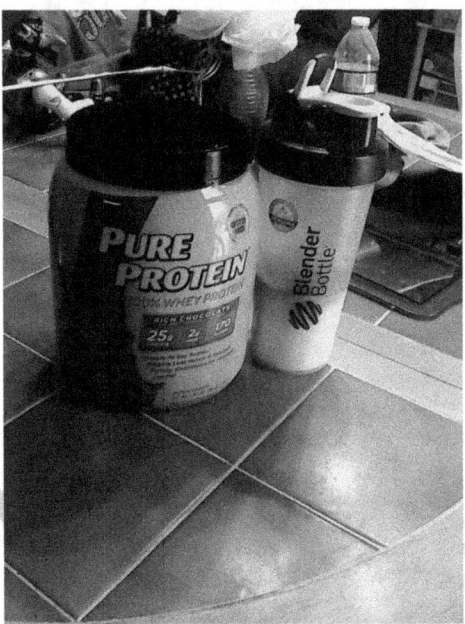

Weight Loss Protein Mix

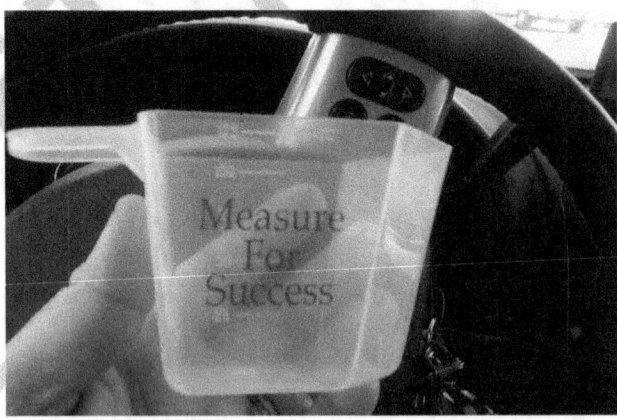

My Pre Op Measuring Cup

Getting Approved

So now that you have completed ALL of the insurance requirements, you are wondering when you will get a surgery date. After you complete each test for the insurance company, your surgeon will request copies of each physicians results. They are building a file to submit to your insurance company. This was the most irritating part of the process for me. Getting approved is the biggest nightmare you will ever face in dealing with insurance companies. My surgeons office faxed all of my completed documentation to my insurance company. I called every single week for almost a month. Initially, they denied me due to needing my PCP to write a handwritten letter on my behalf, correcting documentation and wording from the cardiologist I saw in the pre-op phase, and ICD-10 codes changing. It took six weeks to get this straightened out. I went into this thinking I was getting my surgery right after my pre op appointments ended. I completed those appointments in September 2015.

Then began the waiting game. The waiting game is enough of a stress to cause you more stress than what it's worth. Worrying yourself and continuously calling your surgeon's office will not speed up the process of getting you a surgery date sooner. The surgeon's office cannot do anything for you but keep calling your insurance company for you to find out if you have been approved. I tried calling the insurance company myself but they aren't legally allowed to give you any information on what your surgeon submitted while your case is being reviewed for approval. Your approval will go through a process of two to three people at the insurance company to get approved. Your file will get evaluated by a nurse, a medical physician, and a representative of the insurance company who determines how much insurance will pay or won't pay.

You will spend a lot of time stressed out wondering if you have put in the work for nothing. You will wonder why it is taking so long to get approved. Don't sweat it honey. Give it time. Time is truly all you have. I spent a lot of my time during the waiting game researching over and over my insurance company's requirements again and again to make sure I fit exactly into where they required me to be. When you spend time stressing out about it, you will end up worrying yourself sick. Put your focus on your pre op diet and continue to work on yourself. You have so much to look forward to.

Even if you do get denied, don't give up! Ask for an appeal. If you have to do some more requirements for insurance, don't give up! Just do what you have to do! Your life is at stake! The insurance companies are out to make you go through a heap of paperwork just to get you approved! Most of them don't want to waste paper or time, so they will send you through a mess of requirements just to see if you are willing to follow what they ask of you. Do what you have to do and don't look back!

This was me. I laugh at it now because I know I probably drove my surgeon's office crazy with me calling them daily plus calling my insurance company daily. I guess you could say I was excited and ready to get my surgery done. I already put in my notice at work to be off the first few weeks of September. I kept having to retract my surgery date and it ended up being November 3, 2015. Going back and forth between the insurance company requesting more requirements be met or the paperwork to get fixed caused me to miss a lot of days at work as well. In the end, I guess you could say I was over prepared for my surgery. Each day I would call my doctor or the insurance company just to get a "waiting" response, it would cause negative doubts to cross into my mind. I mostly wondered if everything I had been doing was worth it just for the insurance company to turn me down. I tried to stay positive and keep my mind positive as much as possible. Possibilities and doubts lead to negative thinking and negative outcomes. I kept a low profile as much as I possibly could to keep anyone else's negative thoughts about my upcoming surgery out of my head. My ultimate goal and purpose was to save my life from the death sentence known as obesity. A purpose is dead without motivation and a positive attitude to fuel it. The insurance company finally gave me a decision after almost six weeks. I got the notice from my insurance company before I got the call from my surgeon's office. This made me a little angry, but it is what it is. I was just happy to find out they approved me. I can remember the day I found out. I was sitting outside in my car at work on the phone with my insurance company. The woman had me on hold what seemed like forever. My husband was inside our workplace finishing up his paperwork for the day. The lady finally gets back on the phone and tells me I am approved. I didn't know whether to jump up and down, cry, or run in circles. An immense feeling of peace came over me while I sat outside speechless. After I got off the phone, my boss came outside. She also had weight loss surgery and lost over 200 pounds. I jumped out of the car and ran up to her hugging her, crying, and jumping up and down. I was so excited! Just a sense of relief and peace came over me. She hugged me, congratulated me, and left. I remember walking back to my car and feeling so angry about her support in the beginning but not at the end, that I sat in the car and cried my eyes out. Tears of joy for myself. No tears were shed for her not being happy for me. I knew she didn't care anyways. Ever since I mentioned weight loss surgery, her and others at my job changed their thinking of me. They treated me like crap and were arrogant towards me. Life is like a bus. As you are going along, people are going to get on and get off at random times. Some will bring you joy and be with you rooting you on forever, while others are just there for the ride until they fizzle out on you. At that moment is when it's time to make the decision. It's time to put them off your bus and make room for the ones who actually want to be on the bus with you and help you to succeed. While I was going through the approval process, my coworkers tried to lay seeds of doubt in my mind about my surgery and how it would change the kind of person I am. Truly, they were right. It made me realize who my supporters were and who they weren't. Many times along my weight loss journey, I struggled with figuring out who was for me and against me. In the end, there were very few left standing after I put most of them off of my bus. I became a stronger woman because of them. Without their seeds of doubt, I would not have fought harder to get my surgery done. Don't let others seeds of doubt take root in your life. Do like I did and keep your bus moving full steam ahead.

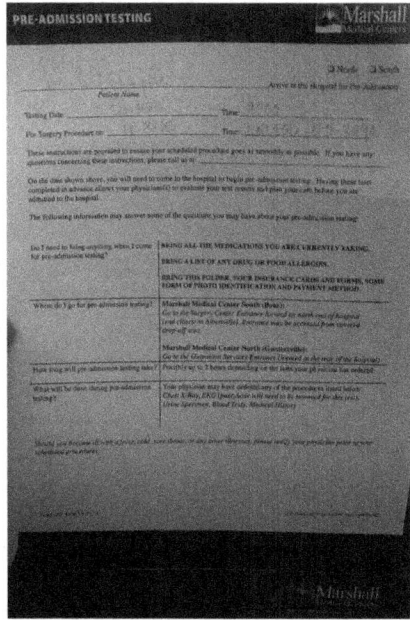

Pre Op Testing

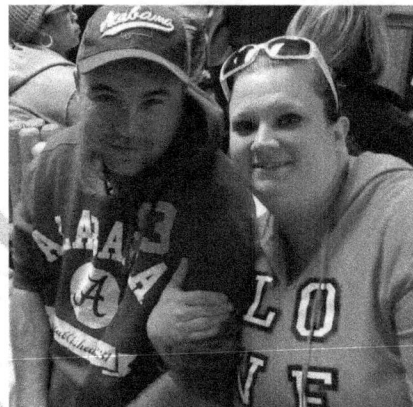

This is me one week before surgery

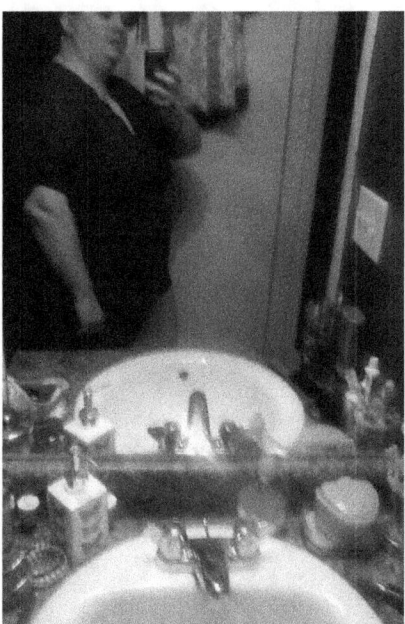

My overhang one week before surgery

Friends Will Come And Go

Between the time you start this entire process up until after you lose your weight, you will have people who were so committed to you losing weight and promising to be there for you throughout the process. When you decide you are going to do the gastric sleeve surgery, the first people you tell are your closest friends and your family. You want them to be excited for you and support you. When you finally reveal to them your decision, you will find quite a few who do not agree with your decision for surgery. You will get comments about going to the gym, to do it the natural way, and then people who suggest you join some diet fad. Harsh reality is that many times, the people who you think support you are really behind you wishing you would fail. Your feelings are going to be hurt. People are going to walk out of your life because you are "taking the easy way out".

Honestly, going through the process just to get the surgery and then the process of recovery after the surgery isn't the easy way out like people think. The time you would have spent at the gym exercising equals about the same time spent as the process of getting the surgery.

In my own personal situation, I was the fat friend. I was the one people invited because I was the heavy one that made them look better. One instance being when I helped coach cheerleading. The other lady always made the comment that I wasn't able to do the stunts. Truth of the matter was that I wasn't really able to, but it wasn't her job to constantly remind me and everyone else there. I was constantly put on the center of attention because I didn't have workout clothes that fit properly or I had to spend the practicing time rearranging my clothes to make them fit and cover me up. Growing up thin, I never had this kind of problem. I was always the friend that attracted attention because people thought I was pretty and had a good body. I was the center of attention for the wrong reasons. People were my friend because I attracted others by my beauty. The real me inside didn't matter to the friends who were only interested in me because of my outer appearance. I was always thin in school. I could eat what I want and not gain a pound up until I had my daughter at 23. As I gained weight, these friends drifted away because I was no longer the thin beauty queen. I passed them in weight and we reversed roles. Role reversal is the problem between you and the people who quit being your friend. You will either have friends who will support you while you are the fat friend and bail on you when you start to attract attention for your weight loss journey or you will have friends who supported you when you were the fat friend and continued to cheer you on while you are on your journey. The one friend I have had throughout this journey is another woman who knew me before surgery was even considered and supports me up until today is a woman who had a weight loss surgery like I did. We have a special bond that has connected us from the beginning when we first met during an Autism rally five years ago (2010). The friends you used to have become just mere acquaintances just like mine.

It has been hard to lose touch with friends I used to go shopping with and work on independent projects with. I have spent many nights and days trying to figure out what I did wrong to them, but truly it wasn't me. The dynamics of our relationship changed. The dynamics of all of the relationships around you change. The relationships of mine that changed were work, close friends, family, and church friends. My relationship with my husband has gotten stronger throughout this process. He has helped me get to where I am now and continues to help me get to where I am going. It did take him some time to get used to the things I was able to eat now. He has even lost some weight along my journey. It took him some time to get used to the changes my body has been experiencing since surgery. As my husband, he has had to take on a lot of extra responsibilities during my recovery time, such as taking care of 4 kids, pets, household chores, and become the breadwinner. He has also had to learn about proteins and the kinds of foods I can eat and has had to help me with a PICC line and other things. My weight loss journey has brought us closer together as we have learned to depend on one another more. My work friends were a different situation.

At my job, before surgery, I was the go to person for new employees in training. I created manuals and wrote descriptions of phone numbers of who to call along with different scenarios to help new employees get started. I also took new employees out on drive around training, introduced them to our local companies, and helped with after hours calls. While I was there helping other people get started with the company, I would constantly get pulled into a conversation with the same boss lady who supported me in the beginning and fizzled out on me in the middle. She would throw a line to me about becoming office staff and then turn around a week later and hire someone else. Then, when they quit, she would run back to me and offer the same position. It was a vicious cycle that finally ended. I was thankful for that because I had gotten tired of being her fall back girl all the time. There comes a time when you get tired of being used. This was that time. During my process leading up to surgery, I started to miss days of work. Everyone at work was okay with me missing days and acted happy about me "getting my life back". When I started giving them less of my time, my "supporters" disappeared. I was a little hurt, but I knew they needed off my support bus. The dynamics at work changed during this time up until I eventually turned in my notice to quit. I had enough of being used and strung along like a puppet. Constantly, pulled in and out of the conversation and offered an office job. Honestly, I have done better by myself and working for myself than I did being someone else's puppet. At the end of my time period there and after coming back and working three more months after surgery, I had made my decision and quit. For all of the people who supported me and gungho for me and promised to always be here and that I will always have a job, they slowly sent me out the door after my surgery because for once I stood up for myself. I got tired of their mess on me. I am happy I left there because they caused me more issues than I needed. They were no longer on my bus going north. They were holding me back from the greater potential I carried inside. Just like my ex coworkers, the dynamics of my close friendships changed. Like I said, I was no longer that fat friend to go shop for fat clothes with. I truly believe our interests changed. I was no longer interested in fad diets, crying in my pity party, or trying to figure out how to get my weight off. I mostly was interested in getting healthy. You find out who you friends are when your appearance changes and you lose weight. For the friends who walked away from me because my interests and focus changed towards myself, God sent true friends my way by means of a new church. Most of my friends were at the church we attended. After my surgery in November, we found a new church home with so many amazing ladies and men to pray for our needs. They have shown me what true friendship means by their actions. If your church family has a negative comment about you taking the surgery route, you know it is time to find a new church home. I just thank God for bringing new people into our lives. God had been preparing His plans for us before we even knew it. He come right in and provided the support I needed as the different groups of people I have had in my life come and go.

Friends will come and go while you go through this process. Some were meant to stay while others were meant to be here temporarily to teach you new ideas above and beyond your wildest imagination. Each person who comes and goes in your life takes away a piece of you while others leave a piece of themselves in your heart. These pieces leave scars and pain in your heart. Eventually, my scars and the pieces former friends left behind were replaced with love, hope, and a promise from God to fill my life with more people. Many times, I have felt alone and needed a friend. These scars are slowly healing from the wounds of obesity. I am such a social butterfly that it bothers me when I am not surrounded by lots of people. I have let go of my dependency factor since my surgery. I used to be co dependent upon others in my time of need or when I needed someone to share my feelings with. Throughout my journey, I have learned to turn my co dependence issue into hobbies, hopes, and dreams. I refocused my thoughts and feelings into reconstructing myself and my life with positive influences. Having a positive outlook and influence helps to heal many of the wounds I still carry from obesity.

Can You See Me?

This is a poem I wrote about my experience and feelings in dressing rooms at different stores. It was always the same feelings but a different store. My feelings now have changed since I have changed. People treat me differently now that they do not see the "fat me" anymore.

Can You See Me?

Can you see me?
I'm the girl standing in line
Patiently waiting on a dressing room
Wondering why you've waited on everyone but me.

I've been standing here
longer than all the others.
What makes me different
Than any of the others?

Do I not fit in?
Do I not belong in this place?
Is it because you only see thin?
How can you walk by
and not see my face?

I deserve to be here like the rest.
All I want is to try on these clothes
And look my best.

Can you see me?
Its been five minutes.
I've stood here like all the rest.
I've watched you walk by
And not acknowledge my presence.
Are you afraid to be honest?
Afraid to face me?
Afraid to just look and see me?

Can you see me?
Waiting on this dressing room
To try on clothes I hope to fit.
I won't be long.
I promise to put away things
That don't fit.

Can you see me?
Am I too big to be shopping here?
Has the fear of losing your job
Or the fear of rejection
Caused you not to see me?

Can you see me?
Are you afraid of having to look my way

Or worse, making eye contact with me?
Can't you see me standing here?
All I want is to be accepted here.
All I want is to be seen,
Heard,
And to hear the words
The words I'm coming to help you.
Instead of being ignored,
Not being seen,
Not being heard,
Not allowed to try on clothes
In a dressing room.

Can you see me?
I've give up waiting on you to let me in,
Waiting on you to notice me,
Waiting on you to see me.

You never even noticed me as I waited
On you to help me.
All you saw was a fat girl
Trying to try on new clothes
And trying to blend in.

Can you see me?
As I hang my clothes on the rack
Outside the dressing room door
Still all I could see was your back.

So I gave you mine.
I made myself fade into the crowd
And acted like I was just fine.
Tryimg to escape the pit inside
The one in my stomach
I always seem to hide.

Did you see me as I left?
I just hung up my clothes
And walked right out.
Maybe next time you see me
You will see a new me.
You will see the one we both can see.
Don't let anyone else walk out
And wonder
Can you see me?

Your Mental Health Before and After The Sleeve

There is so much to describe in the changes before and after surgery. The surgery changes you as a whole person over a gradual period of time. In many ways, I became a better person, while in other ways, I lost parts of myself that hid behind all the fat numbers I carried on my waistline for so long. I lost the parts of me that people laughed with and joked around with. I gained an attitude of self-respect for myself and put down my foot on what I would allow myself to be a part of anymore. People are either going to love you or hate on you. Honestly, their opinion is worthless. The one you should stay focused on is yourself.

Eventually, this will either drive people away from you or bring them closer to you. If you chase away the people who left you during the process, you will wear yourself down and end up feeling like you are losing your mind. The surgery plays tricks on your mind. After the surgery, you will have a hard time sorting out your own feelings much less the feelings of others who are there to put you down.

For myself, before the gastric sleeve, I lived a life of desperation. I lived for other people. I lived for people to like me, to not see the fat I was drowning in, and desperate for friendships. I mean, who wants to have a friend they go shopping with who can't fit into anything cute at the small clothing stores. I was scared to go shopping because I brought home hurt feelings most of the time. Before the surgery, I was desperate for people to like the person I was inside more than the person they seen on the outside. I did my best to distract people from the fat on the outside by making them feel good and a few times making a joke of myself. I was known as the girl who would jump out there and try anything. I did it to hide myself from all the feelings I had inside of myself. For many years I carried the burdens of my family and the divorce I experienced as a teenager. At a time I needed someone the most, I had nobody and was dropped into the foster care system to fend for myself. During my time in the system, I turned to food. Food was my comfort. As long as I fed myself and stuffed myself into misery, I didn't have to worry about pleasing others. I had some weight gain during this time, but not as much as pregnancy in my early twenties. I learned to eat junk food in the foster care system. Not because I wanted to, but because this was all the foster care home had to eat. I lived off of Pop Tarts and Chips. Not once did the foster home woman ever cook a good decent meal for us children. With eight to ten kids there, she should have at least used the welfare money given to her to cook for us and provide us with a good home. I had spent my life with both of my parents. I had grown up in a two parent home, had excellent grades, sports, activities, and both parents provided for us above and beyond, but, when divorce came, my brother and I were left with nothing. Nobody to turn to or ask for help. My brother was 18 and dumped on the street and myself, I was dumped in foster care. I spent my entire life working on keeping good grades, staying out of trouble, and doing the right thing just to end up dropped off in the welfare system. I had no clue how to manage money, get a job, or take care of myself. I used food as my comfort in foster care to hide who I really was. Inside I was screaming to get out of foster care and get my life back. I felt like my life had been ripped out from under me without a rug to sit on much less stand on. I basically had to start from scratch. My bad eating habits came from this time period in my life. I was depressed and would eat until I could no longer feel the pain in my heart for my family dumping me. As I gained weight, I would get even more depressed and eventually would land myself in the mental health center for teens. I would eat and force myself to throw up. I would binge eat and then run to the bathroom at the foster home. Anytime I got called fat or overweight, I would run for a knife at the foster home and try to cut off what I saw as fat on me, when it was really not fat, but just skin over my bony ribs. The view I had of myself was ugly and terrible. I felt to blame for my family falling apart.

My mental health was at its deepest darkest hole during this time in my life. I was overweight (in my mind, not on the scale). I was in a new place with new people I didn't know. I was also struggling with my parents divorce. I turned to food to help submerge some of my wounds. I waited until my 18th birthday and I ended up leaving foster care on my own. I literally had nothing. Nowhere to go and nothing of my own. I was virtually homeless. Before my surgery, I would turn to food and taking mental health pills to ease the scars of my life. If these things had happened to me after surgery, I would probably have been better equipped to handle what life has thrown at me. Excess weight on your body causes stress on your mental health and psychiatric welfare. It causes whatever problems you have been carrying to be multiplied. During my life at this time, I was struggling with so much that I spent a year in the mental health center for teens working to get my life back together and get control of my psychiatric issues. An eating disorder didn't help my overall health situation. Post Traumatic Stress Disorder will also further keep you from keeping weight off. With all of the medications I was on from my mental health issues at the time, weight just kept piling on to my body.

I encourage you, that if you are suffering from the same kind of issues as I have gone through, that you will incorporate exercise into your daily regimen. Before my surgery, I lacked the proper coping skills to help me deal with the issues going on within myself. It was easy to run to food for comfort.

After surgery, my mental health has changed. If I could go back and change things I have went through, I would have reacted differently in my life. Instead of running to food, I would have used those experiences to build my self esteem up as well as prepare myself mentally to deal with the challenges that come with becoming an adult. I do believe that over time, our minds will change and we learn new coping strategies. As we grow into adults and transition into adulthood from teenage years, our minds adjust to stress differently. With the weight gone, I haven't been so bogged down with stress from worrying about my health and other things going on in my life. I don't regret my surgery, but there are times that I do get overwhelmed and have to visit my own "War Room" to have a talk with God. Having a safe place to go to cry your eyes out and get some quiet time is important after surgery. It gives you time to yourself as you transition your life from obesity to healthy. Changing your foods restarts your body and these foods cause changes mentally inside of you. Some of those changes include how you feel about yourself, your self-esteem, how you treat others around you, and how you react to different situations. My best advice is to do your best to work through things slowly and not to expect a quick change overnight. Also, not to lose your temper in a quick response to anger. After surgery, I was a "short fuse" for a while learning how to deal with people differently. People will view you differently after weight loss surgery and you will feel it internally. Finding yourself starts with figuring out who you are and where you are going with your life.

Its Surgery Day!

Today is Your Day

Today you join the famous Loser Bench! You have made it to surgery! What to expect today? Lots of activity and a long journey on your way to a healthy lifestyle.

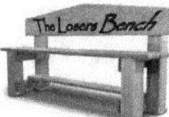

I joined the Loser

The Losers Bench is famous because it represents exactly what you have worked for during your preparation time. This bench is famous for the many others who have come before you and will follow in your footsteps. My "Sleeversary" (Sleeve Anniversary) is November 3, 2015, the day I joined the Losers Bench. My "Sleeversary" will forever be ingrained in my heart because it represents the first day of the rest of my second chance at life God has given me. I thank God for giving me the opportunity to gain my life back again. No doubt, a drastic measure, but definitely worth the risk.

Just like you, I thought I knew it all and had everything planned in my mind. That was until I got to the hospital. I used the Hibiclens given to me a few days before by the hospital staff as well as took all of the necessary precautions to keep myself safe and well. I did not sleep a wink the night before because I was so overcome with nervousness and gratitude. My surgery was scheduled at 10 am. I got into registration that morning at 7:30 a.m. ready to get my day started. My mom, husband, and daughter were with me during my surgery date. After waiting about fifteen minutes, my name was called and I had to kiss my family goodbye to head to the surgery preparation room. They were all hugging me, crying, and praying for me, but I knew God was already in control and had my back. I waved my goodbyes and was wheeled off to my preparation room.

When I got there, my surgeon was waiting on me as well as the rest of the team who would be taking care of me. I got the usual treatment of an IV, monitors, and the gown. My family was allowed to come in after I was connected onto the IV and helped me get dressed in my gown. I was so worried and nervous thinking about my family. I thank God for showing up in the smallest moments and giving me and my family a good laugh in the midst of our worries that day. The room I was in for prep had a toilet that would flush on its own repeatedly even with no one around. Each time maintenance would show up, it would quit. As soon as maintenance left, the toilet would start again. I see it as God sending a sign to get my mind off things worrying us. God replaced our worry with laughter. Sometimes, He will do that. God will use signs to show you things.

I waited for two hours until the nurses came to my pre surgery prep room to take me to surgery. My husband was hugging and kissing me and my mom was crying with worry again. I gave them my thumbs up and my hospital bed was on the move. The nurses took me to the surgery waiting room and went over my last minute details. They explained my surgery once again and asked about taking photos of the specimen my surgery would be removing. Of course, the scientist in me was curious. The photograph below is what I received after surgery. This is the Ghrelin, the portion that controls hunger. It is smaller than I first imagined. I look at this picture when I need a reminder of exactly how big my stomach is now in relation to before surgery. There are times when you have to put things into perspective.

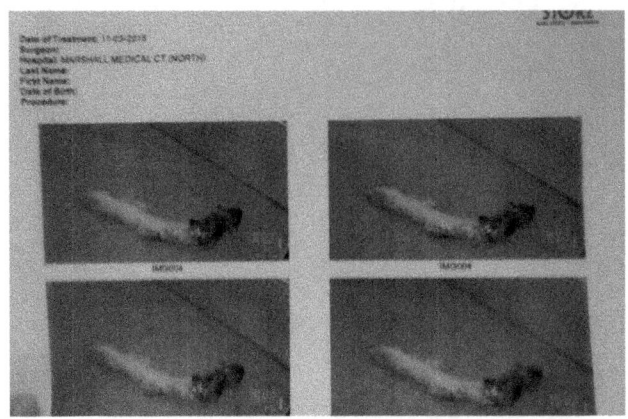

This is the portion of the stomach they remove from you. It is called the Ghrelin.

IT'S MY SURGERY DAY!!!

I did get to speak with my surgeon before surgery. He came into the waiting room and helped to wheel me in and check on my anesthesia. I remember him praying for me and telling me he would see me on the other side. Just forever grateful for him and all he has helped me to accomplish. God used him to save my life. I remember trying to count to ten, but I only made it to 3 before I fell asleep.

Little did I know while I was in surgery, things went well. My surgery lasted about 45 minutes. My surgeon called my family to let them know I was doing well and the surgery was a success. They also told me he came down to my pre surgery waiting room and gave them the details of my surgery as well as thanking them for being here for me.

Surgery Day really wasn't as bad as I expected. More fears than anything else. I am thankful to look back on that day and know that I had a positive experience.

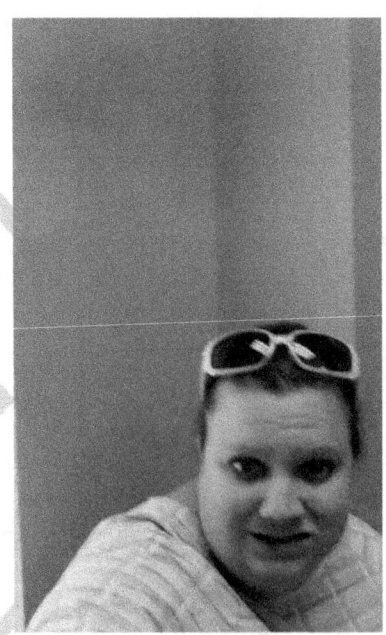

Me Getting Ready to Go In

Recovery And Resting

Recovery from surgery starts immediately and it is important to start taking care of yourself properly as soon as you come out of surgery. The most important advice I can give you is get lots of rest and keep hydrated. There is absolutely no way you will be able to drink a whole 20 ounce bottle of water like before so you will have to sip, sip and sip some more. Your stomach just doesn't have enough room for a whole bottle of water anymore. Personally, I bought a sports cup with the amounts on the side of it so I could keep up with my water intake. You will feel full most of the time and not think much about food. You will need to keep drinking water though. Water is the your best friend on the road to recovery.

When you wake up from surgery, you will be on clear liquids and graduate over the next six weeks to liquids, purees, soft foods, and then regular solids. It will seem like it takes forever to get to where you can start to eat regular food again. Over the next few weeks, you will learn when you are at your point of being full. Your body will give you signs of when you are full. Personally, my stomach pouch would give a simple hiccup. I can't speak personally for myself, so I don't know about others reactions. Your stomach will also hurt in a terrible pain that you will never forget. It feels like you swallowed a balloon. I don't recommend overfilling your stomach pouch. You will make yourself sick. Eat small portions. Sip small sips.

Much of your recovery will depend on how much rest you get. You won't get a lot of sleep due to every time you move around in bed or while you are sitting upright, you will feel small tinges of pain from your incisions. My incisions only hurt me for about two weeks. Most of my pain came from laying in my bed at night. I had to stuff my back and around my abdomen with a long body pillow to kind of hold my body in one place while I slept on my back. My family most of the time stayed mad at me for sleeping on my back because I was unable to just jump up and run to their aid like they were used to. Ignore them and focus on yourself. For me, the best way to get rest was to sit up straight in my recliner with my back stuffed with pillows around it. Do what makes you comfortable. I wasn't able to even get up and move around a lot, so don't expect to be able to do that either.

You need your recovery time regardless of how anyone else feels. I slept for many hours during the day. I didn't need people to help me with anything at home except for some light housework, like mopping and doing laundry. I wasn't able to lift or pick up anything over five pounds for almost a month. I needed light help with taking a shower as it was hard to lift my legs up over the side of the bathtub to get in. I also wrapped my incisions with a plastic shopping bag to keep them from getting wet. Coming home was the easy part. The first two days home were the worst as I was trying to get used to the changes I had experienced and continuing to experience.

Each day gets easier. I noticed my weight dropping immediately when I got home. They say you should stay off the scale. Not for me! The scale was my motivation! Each morning it was a game just to see how much weight I had lost since the day before. It turned out to be a great project for me. It helps to see that you are making progress and getting somewhere. Without a scale, you don't know if your numbers are going in the right direction or not. Within a week, I had to send my clothes to Goodwill. Most did not fit anymore and my precious sundresses went as well.

Coming Home

I spent one night in the hospital and came home the next day. Waking up from surgery, I was sick and nauseous. I was in incredible pain, but I kept telling myself "It's worth it". There wasn't really any prep the morning of surgery, other than the Hibiclens I had to shower with. When I got into admissions at the hospital, I was basically brought into surgery prep and given an IV. I had to put on my hospital gown as well. Many things stick out in my mind that morning as I was waiting to go back for surgery. My mom and my husband were there along with my daughter. Looking back, I know that God had me in that room for a purpose. It was to give me a laugh to calm my nerves a little. I was a nervous wreck and more excited than scared. I don't remember being scared at all. I was just excited because my day had finally come. I spent most of the morning wondering how I would do after surgery coming home. I mean, you read all of these horror stories and problems that others had after surgery hoping and praying that you won't be one of those people you heard about. Laughter was certainly provided for me and my family that morning. God will show up when you least expect him to calm you when you are in the biggest storms of your life.

That morning, my family and I sat in my pre-surgery room waiting for the doctor to wheel me in to surgery. I had gotten up three times out of my hospital bed going back and forth to the restroom in my room. Each time I come out of the restroom, the toilet would reflush itself multiple times. It would constantly do this over and over again. My mom called the janitor and maintenance man, who came to my room and the toilet would stop itself. Each time he would show up, the toilet would stop. When he left the room, it would start up again. As my time drew closer to be wheeled back into surgery, my family and I would laugh and laugh because it was ironic how during your times of worry and stress, God would show up and provide you with some laughter to get you through these times. Finally, my time had come and as I was wheeled down the hall, I shed tears of joy because I know my laugh was about to change. Tears rolled down my eyes until I fell asleep.

When I awoke, like I said I was in so much pain. The pain after the gastric sleeve surgery is comparable to having a Cesarean Section, except you can actually stand up. When I stood up, I felt my insides moving around and they felt like they would fall out of me. My stomach had been cut out 90% and I was left with a small banana shaped portion. My stomach only held half a cup of food, but the last thing on my mind was food. During the surgery, my surgeon had cut out the portion of my stomach that controls hunger, called the Ghrelin. It controls hunger hormones and sends signals to your brain and body that you are hungry. Waking up from surgery, I was put on a liquid diet to keep my stomach under control and give it time to heal from the surgery. To be honest, the last thing on my mind was food. I didn't feel hungry or feel like eating anything.

I had to drink so much water to stay hydrated. I couldn't get enough water when I got home. I can remember living off of liquids from soup and jello. The first phase of eating when you come home is liquids. I had to stay on liquids for two weeks. At first, I didn't think I could live off liquids, but after coming home and feeling like I couldn't eat anything, I quickly realized I had no choice but to force myself on the required liquids to stay alive. The first week home, I lost over 20 pounds. The equation works like this: the smaller your stomach, the smaller the portion it will hold=the less calories you take in and the more weight you lose. Simple equation, yet complicated to wrap your mind around. As humans, we are so used to eating way above our portion size and when we are forced to eat less, it will take some time to get used to.

The things I am grateful for buying before surgery helped me so much when I came home from surgery. Many of these things you will want to invest in yourself before surgery. The best thing I ever purchased was my long body pillow. I bought a long round one that my whole body could lay on. It became my best friend while I was at home recovering from surgery. I would twist it and turn it around different positions to hold up the portions of my body I felt like were falling inside when I moved. Just like after having a baby, your insides will shift around to figure out exactly where they "sit" again inside of your tummy. My pillow spent most of its time wrapped around my ribs as this was the first place for me to lose my body weight. Even now, six months after surgery, I can't lay on my sides because my ribs feel like they are getting smashed in. The second best thing I bought before surgery was a shaker cup. I bought my shaker cup at Kroger. It has a metal ball inside that helps to mix up my protein shakes better. My surgeon was a little different than other surgeons I know of. He encouraged proteins, but protein intake coming from food instead of protein shakes. The first week home, I got proteins from liquid soups and different foods I had to eat.

The second phase when I came home was pureed foods. This included mashed potatoes, mashed peas, yogurt, and mashed bananas. This was the hardest for me. There just comes a time when you are exhausted from eating the same soups and food over and over again. Peanut Butter was still a no on the list of foods I couldn't eat because of the fear of it sticking to the insides of my stomach. I didn't crave foods like I used to before the surgery. I spent a lot of my time during the first phase and second phase (approximately a month) laying in bed recovering and trying to make myself comfortable. The best thing I could do for myself was to make myself comfortable because the pain was so unbearable at times. I could no longer take pain medication or any medication for that matter. The composition of your stomach changes and your entire life and way of eating changes. Your mindset changes. When you get home, all you want to do is rest and start working on the plans God has had buried in your heart underneath all the weight you used to carry. When you finally start to feel better after coming home, you start to find yourself in position where you are waking up at 4 am fired up and ready to run a mile. The mental drain and anguish you used to feel have subsided and you begin to feel such an empowerment to get out and do the things in life that the weight held you back from. These thoughts kicked in for me during my third phase of recovery.

The third phase of recovery is soft foods. The foods in this category include lots of tuna fish, chicken cut up into small pieces, and protein filled dairy like cottage cheese. I was so glad to get to this phase. By this time, I was in my fifth and sixth week of recovery. The soft food phase lasts about two weeks. At my fifth and sixth week check in, I had lost almost 45 pounds. My clothes and attitude changed too. My family started noticing my changes, mostly my face thinning out and my clothes were way too big. The soft food phase was tricky for me at times. I started to take a step out here and there to try new foods. I tried foods and fruits I have never eaten before. Cantaloupe became my obsession. I couldn't get enough of cantaloupe. Grocery shopping became fun and I thank God for my mom coming along and helping me pick out foods I could eat. It wasn't easy, but it definitely was a challenge. Soft foods come into play when your taste buds regain hunger. To satisfy my taste buds, there were many times I would drink gallons of water. Gallons of water were exactly what my body needed to keep me healthy. Some of the underlying conditions I had before surgery were related to confusing thirsty signals with hunger signals. My body was actually thirsty for water and not actually hungry for food. Distinguishing the difference will become a challenge as you try to separate the truth from the signals in your body playing tricks on you. Now that my Ghrelin was gone and taken out from surgery, I know my idea of hungry was just in my head. To keep yourself from eating out of boredom and eating because you need something to do, you will have to do like me and find yourself a form or way of therapy. Mine just happened to be writing this book. This book has become my way of healing myself and healing the scars from my past that were hid underneath all of the weight I carried with me for so many years.

Coming home was the toughest possible thing I have ever done in my life. This surgery has been one of the toughest things in my life I have ever had to endure. Sometimes God will give you the hardest things to endure to make you the strongest warrior on the field. This is that battle for me. Coming home to a new life and a new experience has changed the way I look at my life. When I first come home after surgery, I felt sick and just lethargic. I wondered why I chose this, but in the end I have no regrets. If I could go back and change the way I lived my life before surgery, I would do things differently. Coming home gives you a new perspective on things. The way you view yourself and the way you carry yourself changes. The way you treat yourself during the first three phases of coming home determine how well you will do when you finally start to eat normal foods.

Eating normal foods is different now. My description of normal isn't the same as before. Before my surgery, my description of normal foods was popcorn chicken, fries, nuggets, huge sandwiches, fried foods, and fast food. These foods were actually the reason I ended up overweight and my body in the mess it was in. These were my comfort foods. These were the only foods I had virtually known my whole life, plus a few more including hot dogs and chips. Coming home, I no longer craved these foods. I craved healthy whole foods, like carrots, beans, lentils, and tuna. My idea of normal foods now is way different than beforehand. Normal foods now for me are tuna, baked chicken, baked fish, no fast food, and beans rich in proteins. Coming home, I realized quickly that I had a new pouch, as we call it in the gastric sleeve community. My "pouch" was lactose and any kind of milk products made me sick. My "pouch" just wouldn't tolerate any kind of milk or dairy products. For the proteins I needed from dairy and milk products, I bought cottage cheese (which actually isn't that bad even though it sounds terrible), mozzarella, and ricotta cheese. During the last phase of coming home, I engaged myself into cooking many different meals that were on my diet. Although my family was a little hesitant at first, they all eventually came around and actually enjoyed some of my recipes. Many times they never even knew that I had substituted their favorite foods for what my new pouch would injest. Looking over the last six months, I have enjoyed my journey of learning new experiences and tasting new food choices that I never would have had the opportunity to do before if I hadn't had the gastric sleeve surgery.

During the time between starting the last phase at eight weeks after surgery up until now, six months later, I have maintained my weight loss journey. I have continued to lose weight and keep up with my eating habits daily. Weight loss is a daily lifelong journey. It doesn't happen overnight and it certainly isn't a quick journey. Starting with eating right is the beginning of the start to my new life. Coming home was a journey in itself, in I had to learn what to eat, when to eat, and how to portion out my food. Learning your body signals is the main way to know that you are full. When I first came home, when I was full my "pouch" would "burp". Now I can tell I am full by how it feels as I am eating. Three main things I encourage you to buy before surgery to get you through the first six months are: long body pillow, shaker cup with a ball, and half plates (kid size) for portion control. These will be your keys to helping you achieve your weight loss goals when you come home.

Top 5 After Surgery Activities To Stay Focused

Top 5 After Surgery Activities To Stay Focused

1. Find a Hobby.

Find something new to do to keep your mind off food and becoming dependent upon food again. For me it has been reading books. Reading books has helped me overcome the struggle during boredom eating. Find a hobby you enjoy and pour your heart into it. Instead of spending money on fast food, invest it in your hobby.

2. Exercise

Exercising and walking helps free your mind of anything bothering you. Exercise releases hormones in your body that make you happy. I am back to doing what I enjoyed in school, which was swimming. Not only does it help clear my mind, but it helps to get me towards my goal of getting my body toned and in shape.

3. Write a Book About Your Journey.

Writing a book has become my way of self help for myself. I am my own counselor and writing has helped me work through so much during my life change from obesity to getting my life back. Always find a professional counselor. Writing has just helped me put my feelings into words on paper.

4. Take A Family Vacation.

After my surgery, I needed time to get away from everyone to have some special family time. I took my husband for a weekend at Hilton Head Island, SC. We had a great time enjoying one another and discovering new places. An adventure is sometimes the cure. The second trip, we took our children on Spring Break to The Rocky Mountains in Colorado. Seeing God's beauty helped give me a new perspective after my surgery. The last trip, we took our family to Manasota Beach in Florida. Sand in your toes feels so good, but the best part was spending time together gathering seashells.

5. Make A List of Things You Weren't Able To Do Before That You Want To Be Able To Do. Create Your Bucket List.

This is probably one of the most important activities. When you gather and form your ideas onto one sheet of paper you put your focus in focus. You create a picture and list of where you are going. My bucket list includes: Hilton Head Island, Tybee Island, Rocky Mountains, Swim, Participate in my Kids Sports, Skydive, Run a 5K, Write my Book of my Journey, wear a bathing suit again, and many more. As you can see, some I have completed and others I am still working towards.

I Encourage You To Rediscover Yourself And Find New Opportunities For Your New Life

The World Around Me

The world around me has changed since I first started my journey. The things that used to bother me, like my OCD to keep things clean, my desires for trying out different restaurants, constantly being in the bed sleeping half of the day away, and going out to the dance club no longer exist for me anymore. All of the weight I carried around had given me the attitude of "I don't care because I'm already fat" has been suddenly been replaced with the attitude of "I'm changing my life". A similar transformation has happened inside of me that is more important than anything the outside world could ever give me. That transformation is my heart. My heart sees, feels, and views the world differently. My eyes have been awakened to so much that I have missed out on in life when I was overweight. No longer do I have to miss out on carnival rides because the seat was too small for me. I no longer have to miss out on walking around the neighborhood with my daughter and dog, and most of all I no longer have to miss out on my daughters active lifestyle. She is going places in her soccer career at 8 years old. I am finally to the point in my recovery (six months out) that I can go outside and kick the ball with her. Before surgery, my world existed on the sidelines as far as being active on the soccer field with her. My world has changed so much that at times I wonder how I could have missed so much.

Some of the things that you think are going to break you will actually make you. I had in my mind that I would be helpless for many months after my surgery. I was so wrong. I was up and going within two to three weeks. At three months out< I was finally able to play outside with my daughter. I have noticed a change in her since my surgery as well. She would never ask me to get up and go outside to do things. For many years she saw me struggle with high blood pressure, a stroke, and seizures. All of these things even exacerbated my health issues. My heart would be crushed when I had to sit on the sidelines and watch her do things without me. Now that I am 7 months past surgery, I am able to do things with her that we both never thought I would be able to do.

Along with physical changes in my body, I also had mental changes that caused me to change my daily habits. I used to be hard to wake up every morning and I was grouchy. Since surgery, I am awake at 4 am ready to get the day started. I have so much energy that I feel like I could run a marathon sometimes. To soothe this energy, I have found activities early in the morning to do to get my day started. I start out getting my housework done. I have just enough time between getting myself up and getting up my kids to get my housework done. This has freed up my day to see my chiropractor, family physician, and get some time in for exercising. The old me would get up at 4 am to pee and then crawl back to bed to oversleep. With all of this weight gone, I have undergone so many physical changes that have affected my body. This was one of them.

The world around me changed during my transition. I used to be self conscious about myself. It was enough of an issue that I refused to go inside stores to shop, refused going swimming with my kids, and refused to get out and pump my own gas. Why? It seems stupid but I feel it has to be said. First of all, my clothes didn't fit properly, I was so self conscious about my overhang (muffin top), and I was so uncomfortable. Being uncomfortable in your own clothes and skin is one of the worst feelings you can experience in your life. Every activity I did, including walking in the grocery store, caused my blood pressure to raise up to stroke levels. I constantly had to keep pulling my pants up over my overhang and the crotch of my pants and capris never fit properly. Mostly, the world around me didn't change. I changed in the world around me. While everyone else had walked out of my life due to my upcoming surgery and my change in appearance and attitude, I had become so focused on myself and my health that I lost interest in what others were doing in my immediate circle of friends and family. After surgery, I just kind of showed back up and people just stared at me trying to comprehend my physical changes on the outside, while I was sorting out the changes going on inside of myself. Others in my life told me I made them miserable. Truly, I feel I made them miserable because I was no longer their doormat or "fat friend" to dump their problems onto.

No doubt, I did my best to love on them and overlook their faults, I still knew that God had control of the situation. God always has control of the situation and He will never give you more than you can handle at one time. While I have felt like others bailed on me before and during my transition period, I realize now that God truly had my best interests at heart because the people back then couldn't handle me now. I have learned to take control of my situation and eating. I have learned to take responsibility for myself and not depend on others for my success. I am a changed person inside and out. Getting a new start has helped me to realize how much God has taken care of me and where He has brought me from. A lot of my fears and anxiety of the world around me have subsided since surgery. When you change your life, the world around you changes. I try to keep this in mind as my journey continues and more people step on and off my travelling bus in my life. I used to take things personally and would spend days contemplating how I was wrong or wondering what I did wrong, but truly I wasn't to blame. I am no longer to blame for how the world treats me now or how the world treated me in my past. Once I got to the point of this acceptance, I began to rebuild my life and move on. The world around me changed from me being the one to blame to me deciding that my reaction to the rest of the world would forever change.

After surgery, my scenery changed. I ended up going back to my job for about three months only for it to end because I had realized I had moved on from the people and the job I had left behind before my surgery. Going back to work put more stress on me than what it was worth, so I invested in myself. I started working towards my lifelong goals of owning my own business. My husband and I started a Pilot Car and Transport business of our own and I became one of the ladies you hear about that work from home. This transition to working at home has helped me to gain better insight into my future. It helped me to learn to control my eating habits as well as ensured that I was taking the appropriate steps toward my after care.

Being a stay at home worker also allowed me to focus on my family. I am able to stay at home and take care of my well being as well as my children. The road to recovery lasts years. The world may be moving around me, but my outlook on the world is different. Having the surgery gave me such a sense of empowerment. It empowered me to take a step forward in the direction of owning my own few businesses as well as focusing on my husbands business. Most of my recovery has been at home. Being in familiar surroundings and having time to focus on my needs, desires, goals, and wants has helped me to get where I am going in my future.

Since surgery, I no longer fear getting out of the car to pump gas, get groceries from inside a store, or doing things outside with my children. I no longer see the world as a threat to my mentality or a threat to my mental health. I no longer see people's opinion as a fear. The only thing to fear is fear itself. If I spent my life fearing what others had to say about me or cared about their opinions, I wouldn't be where I am now. I feel so confident in my skin now without fear of rejection or gossip about how my clothes fit on me or my weight or my figure at the swimming pool. I am no longer a victim of my weight or my body. I have so much left to accomplish in life and in the world. All I truly want to do with this book is to make a difference in someone else's life. I want to reach out of these pages and give them a hug to let them know that they are not alone in their journey and struggle. I want everyone I meet and come into contact with to be inspired to look outside of your comfort zone and ignore what the world has accustomed you to be comfortable in and grab a hold of all life has to offer you.

The sleeve gastrectomy was a new chance to see the world around me and find myself at the same time. I have rediscovered myself and the world around me by letting go of the past and looking towards my future. The world is a cold and cruel place to you when you are overweight. The constant comments at the store were more noticeable when I was overweight. Or worse, is experiencing someone ignoring you as you wait on a dressing room. The opinion of the world around me doesn't matter at this point. The only person I have to please is God. If anything has came out of my journey, I have gotten a closer relationship with God and learned to pray. I used to pray for the world around me to accept me. Now I pray for me to accept the world around me and to look at overweight people with love. I hope to reach my hand out to the world and make a difference by teaching others to embrace one another instead of being so judgmental about the way people look.

The world around me notices me differently now that I have lost so much weight. I used to get noticed and hear negative comments. Now people I don't know stare at me for my hanging skin sometimes. Men notice me now because, all of a sudden, I am thin and pretty. Suddenly, I fit the profile of society's acceptance. When I was overweight, I was ignored, mistreated, and called fat names. Now that I fit society's acceptance of beauty, people want to be my friend, ask me to go shopping, and men stare at me while asking for dates. If society didn't like me thin, then why bother trying to holler at me now. It does hurt my feelings sometimes, but it is something that just has to be accepted and moved forward with. Harping and dwelling on these issues that I cannot control only makes my situation worse. I have learned to ignore these things. I have a husband and certainly not interested in another man, first and foremost. It really irks me that in our society, people have built up such walls of discrimination against people who are obese. This non acceptance of obese people has brought me to where I am now. Everyday I am struggling with the question of how people can be so cruel?

When the role is reversed, things are different. The world around me has such a long way to go to accepting people who don't fit society's view of beautiful. Beauty is in the eye of the beholder. Beauty should be the first thing society sees in everyone. Sadly, this is just a fallacy. Struggling with finding who I am and being accepted are no longer a part of my life because I am who I am. I am perfect in God's eyes. The rest of the world is the one with the problem.

Deciding to have weight loss surgery was one of the biggest decisions of my life. I didn't do it to please the rest of the world. I did it to save my life. Changing my outer appearance was just a part of the journey. Finding myself on the inside was the blessing. Just because others see you differently than how you see yourself doesn't mean you have to listen to them. You determine your own happiness. Let the world change around you, but keep on being you.

Your Outer Appearance, Your Inner Self

My outer appearance has struggled with my inner self for years, over half of my life. It is human nature to try and fix your outside because you don't feel good about yourself on the inside. Before surgery, I would spend so much time trying to get rid of my jelly rolls around my waistline or judge myself against other women. The only real judge of yourself is you. This was a hard concept for me to learn, but eventually I put the pieces together. Before I had my weight loss surgery, my outer appearance used to try and keep up with my inner self. This just isn't possible. I finally learned that for my outer appearance to shine like my inner self, I had to work on getting some things straightened out. Taking responsibility for my weight has been the greatest feat of this process. Before surgery, I struggled with a beautiful person inside screaming to get out of the fat body I was trapped in. I would get passed up for great jobs that I was overqualified for because of my obesity. I would get passed up on other great opportunities because I didn't fit the exact profile of beautiful on the outside. My beautiful person inside was just looking for that one chance, that opportunity, to do something great for others. I wanted to reach outside of myself and help others. I was seeking more fulfillment in my life, but always held back by my weight. Breaking the chains surrounding my body was all I wanted to do. I have always felt like my weight has been something holding me back from what I was destined to do in my life.

My destination in life wasn't over during my weight loss journey. My destination is just beginning. From the moment I woke up from my surgery, I knew my life had been forever changed. When I got home, I lost so much weight the first week home that I had to start sending my fat clothes to the goodwill stores because none of them fit anymore. As my body has changed over the last 7 months, I have had to let go of clothes I used to HAVE to wear because nothing else fit properly. Now I don't HAVE to wear anything. I have a choice. I can finally wear what I WANT to wear for the day instead of what I HAVE to wear. When I was forced to wear the clothes that didn't fit, my inner self was struggling so bad with trying to figure out who I was and why I was in the shape I was in. Obesity hurts your feelings and everyday was a struggle for me. Walking around constantly having to pull up my pants over my muffin top was so embarrassing. My inner self wanted to bust out of my fat clothes and force my body into shorts and jeans. Speaking of jeans, I put on my first pair in over 7 years when I was 3 months post op from my surgery. It felt so good to put on a pair of jeans. My mind was soaring that day as I stood in the mirror in my bathroom and cried. Many times I have stood in my mirror and cried at the clothes I has saved for so long to try and get my body back into. Even more tears were shed as after only being able to wear these clothes for two weeks and then having to send them to goodwill because they were so big on me. My closet has had times of being empty from having throw out literally everything and start all over. This is the kind of thing that causes your self esteem to go sky high. My inner self still looks in the mirror and sees the fat on my body. This is probably always going to be a struggle for me. If being overweight is all you have seen in 8 years, it is the norm for you.

This was my normal. Inside I have struggled with seeing myself as a new person at times. Seeing people who wouldn't give me a chance to try on clothes at my favorite stores really irks me because now that I am thin, they treat me differently.

My outer appearance has had drastic changes. My hair started falling out at 3 months post surgery. My hair was long and naturally curly before surgery. It was thick and hard to manage as well as required all kinds of hair treatments to keep it maintained. I really noticed my hair falling out in the shower more than ever before. I have been using Biotin enriched shampoos and other nutrient rich hair products. Eventually, I had to go get my hair cut and trimmed because it became so uneven and unmanageable. I feel like I have lost a part of me by cutting my hair shorter. There are times you just have to do what you have to do. My hair is balding in spots when I was 7 months post op. I can run my fingers through my hair and put it in a ponytail, but that ponytail is so small that a ponytail holder has to be a kid size. My luscious thick hair is now dry, dead, and frizzy. I have tried to put products in it to give it some life. It is still dead though. My once naturally curly hair is now straight and lacks volume. I hope to one day regain the hair that I lost. Until then, I am doing the best I can do with what I have to work with.

My outer appearance has also changed because my thighs and legs are so thin. My mom calls me "chicken legs" because with the hair loss and the weight loss, they are so thin and hair doesn't grow on my legs anymore. My face has aged some. My skin is pale and ashy at times. I had to change my makeup colors as well as my face regimen at night. My feet have lost so much weight that I have went from a size 11 to a size 8 in shoes. My feet lost weight and Plantar Fasciitis is no longer an issue. I can get up in the mornings and walk without assistance. My heel pains are non existent now. I can go outside and walk my neighborhood with my family without getting exhausted. I no longer have to ride the electric scooter at the grocery store. I feel comfortable enough to get out of my car and go inside to pay for gas. I am comfortable enough to put on a swimsuit and go swimming with my kids. My outer appearance has changed so much since surgery that my inner self has gained the confidence to do things I haven't been able to do before. I have overcome many of these fears that used to hold me back.

When I see the outer me now, I see happiness. I see a new me. I no longer see a double chin that used to sweat when I walked. I no longer see such a huge overhang (muffin top). My clothes fit better and it feels good to be noticed for positive changes instead of negative. People that don't know I had surgery will joke around that I can afford to gain a few pounds. In my mind, I am dying to tell them "No!' There are times when you want to tell people you had surgery and give them some hope. There are other times when you feel it is best to keep your mouth shut. I have messed up a few times and had to hear the same message about how dangerous the surgery is. I want people to know that there are people out here who have had the surgery and doing quite well. When I see photos of the old me, I am disgusted, yet thankful at the same time. Thankful to be alive and well to give others hope.

My advice for anyone going through this life change is to stick with it and focus on yourself. God is going to give you what you need when you need it.

Jumping Over the Stumbling Blocks

Now don't get me wrong, my surgery has been a great "tool", but I have had my fair share of issues since surgery. I haven't had as many issues as others. During my second month after surgery, I developed a Urinary Tract Infection (UTI). I was in constant pain for days. I tried cranberry juice (Diet) and also tried hot tea (non sweet). Nothing helped. I ended up having to go to my family physician. She put me on a medication that was sulfur based (Sulfamides).

I went home hoping to get some relief. You see, after surgery, I was no longer able to take regular medications, like in capsule form or in tablet form. My stomach just doesn't have the capabilities to process and break them down. I took the medication for three days and my condition wasn't getting any better. I was sick to my stomach and running a fever. My husband had to take care of me each time I got nauseaus and hung over the toilet throwing up.

After not being able to hold down any liquids for a day, he called my family doctor. She called in another prescription in powder form.

Insurance issues came up once again for me. After waiting three days for the pharmacy to get a response whether insurance was going to pay or not, i got a notice in the mail where the powder form was denied. Keep in mind that I was still in pain and sick. I appealed there decision and still received a denial. I was at a loss trying to figure out what to do. I know I needed my medication, but I couldn't afford the $800 bill for the medication without my insurance covering it. After appealing twice, I had to call my family physician back. She informed me two days later that I had to go on a PICC line, which is receiving medications by IV form. Within two hours, I was at the hospital getting it inserted. Being my first time getting a PICC line, I didn't know what to expect. I took my mom and family once again with me.

Basically, the PICC line goes into your arm near your heart and it is a straight IV line to your veins and heart to distribute medication in liquid form. A PICC line is also used for other medical reasons as well. The PICC line was worse than the pain after my surgery. With a PICC line, I didn't get put to sleep for it to be inserted. It is done in same day procedures CATH lab. It took almost an hour to be numbed and inserted. After it is inserted, I was taken back to my recovery room where my family was waiting on me. After the PICC line was inserted, I had to wait for 30 minutes for the medications to go through my veins to make sure I didn't have any kind of reaction. At this point, I was in terrible pain and hurting in my arm. I could barely move it around.

Fear was also a part of my trials that day. Not knowing what was next or what to expect kept me from putting my mind on more positive things to come. I basically had a cord connected directly to my heart through my veins in my arm. It was simply an IV. It hurt and burned. Most of all, it was annoying. When I finally got home that evening, home health was at my house to deliver my IV medications and teach me how to take care of myself. I'm usually not one to depend on others, but this time I had to depend on my husband to shower me, wash my hair, do housework, and look after the kids. It was a lot of stress for our house. My husband and I had to give myself the IV medications every 8 hours. It was an hour process to prep, give meds, and clean up afterwards. We did make it those two weeks with the help of family, friends, and God. Within a two month period, I had to get a PICC line done twice. I had to go through the same process twice. The thought of a PICC line evokes a feeling in me of fear. I dread the mention of a PICC line now.

Each time I get sick and need medication, my PCP refers me back to a PICC line to get medications by IV. After the gastric sleeve surgery, you will see there aren't many medications you take that your body will absorb properly. Many of the medications doctors will prescribe you are coated tablets. Your new stomach cannot absorb these medications and they can make you sick sometimes. There is a long list of medications that will eat the lining of your new stomach as well. It's best to get a metabolic panel done each month after surgery until your body has time to adjust to the changes you have undergone.

Blood work, vitamins, and nutrients are vital to your health after surgery. I had issues with anemia and it took a long time to figure out what was wrong with me. Eating the right foods after your surgery will help keep you on track. Anemia can reveal itself as many different other medical issues and can cause you to be misdiagnosed with something else. I thought my blood sugar was low throughout my first few months of surgery, but it was really anemia that I didn't know I had at the time. When my doctor finally figured it out, I had to change some things within my diet to help me with my anemia. This included diet changes and exercise. Anemia has also cause me issues with my monthly cycle. Anemia can cause excessive bleeding as well as issues with pregnancy. I am currently 9 months post op from surgery and 10 weeks pregnant. My first trimester has been spent in and out of the doctors office for bleeding issues. Luckily, I am doing okay and my baby is fine. I am looking to have a successful pregnancy and am under excellent care.

Many of the stumbling blocks after surgery are minor bumps in the road that will eventually disappear on their own. Many of the health issues I experienced right after surgery are non existent now. They are completely gone and other issues, such as pregnancy have appeared. Pregnancy is a major stumbling block and risk right after surgery. I suffered from PCOS (Poly Cystic Ovarian Syndrome) for 8 years before I had my gastric sleeve surgery. I am one those women who never thought they would be able to get pregnant again due to health issues. After losing my weight and having surgery, I got pregnant 4 months after my surgery, but it ended shortly with a miscarriage due to complications within my body from my surgery. I had no idea I was even pregnant until I went to the Emergency Room one night sick with a fever. I spent 5 weeks miscarrying during this pregnancy and, with my Anemia, it only made my miscarriage worse. Shortly after my miscarriage, I got pregnant fifteen days later on June 15th 2016 and finally I had a viable pregnancy. I am on bed rest for the first trimester due to issues related to my weight loss surgery, but over time, these stumbling blocks will be a thing of the past. Each day, I am getting closer to having a healthy pregnancy. I understand now why weight loss surgeons suggest at least 2 years after surgery before attempting pregnancy. There are just so many things that could go wrong and endanger your health at this point in your recovery. My advice for health issues and stumbling blocks you will encounter along the way is to keep in touch with your physician and medical team. They can help you with your health issues more than reading Google online or listening to others.

Recovering From The Past, Uncovering The Real You

Recovering from the past and uncovering the real you is about looking back at where you were when you were at the happiest point in your life and discovering the future that lies ahead of you. Like me, I'm sure you have scars that need to be healed from where you have missed out on so much in your life after the weight gain. Before my weight gain, I was 125 pounds and enjoyed swimming. I was on a swim team most of my life, but after the weight started piling on, my hopes and goals and dreams of swimming professionally faded away. I gained so much weight that the breathing techniques I was accustomed to doing in the water as I swam, became a risk on my life. I would get high blood pressure attacks and my heart would feel like it was going to explode at times. My body was so overweight that I could no longer keep up with my teammates. I used to be the fastest one in the pool and quickly became last place. It hurt my feelings so much to know that I was no longer capable of doing the things I have been accustomed to doing in the past.

Many of the other things I enjoyed became a chore. Simple things, like taking care of myself, became a task and a chore as well. When I was thin, I was a social butterfly. I had so much going on for me and my future. I felt like I was going places. I had my life planned out for me. As I gained more weight, these goals and dreams faded away. Although I had the college credentials, every job interview I went on led to failure. There are so many employers seeking thin and beautiful women to fulfill job roles, but ignore good people who deserve the same opportunity, but are overweight. Jobs and employers mostly seek people that are accepted by the general public. The public in general doesn't like fat people. Fat and overweight people get passed over for good jobs even if they have the right credentials because of society's generalized idea of overweight people. I feel like I have been scarred many times for being overweight. I have felt like I deserved certain jobs, but got skipped over due to weight issues. It has taken me many years to get over these kind of things and certainly have affected the way I judge employers. Now that I am thin, I attract more attention when I apply for jobs. I notice the way recruiters view people who are larger than me. In the back of my mind, I am thinking "If they only knew me a year ago". It's horrible to think this way, but after years of being singled out for my weight, I feel terrible for the ones who don't get chosen for the job.

Everything in life that you embark on is like a job interview. You set yourself up for it. You get dressed up for your plans. Then you appear for the show to begin. The next part is left in the hands of others. You have to hope and wish for the best. Many times what you are hoping for doesn't go your way, but if you are lucky, it will. I feel like having a not so perfect figure is one factor counting against you. Being on stage daily happens when you walk into a store, school, church, and other public places. In your mind, all you can think of is how everyone is judging you and your weight, even if they are not. It is hard to change your mindset after surgery to figure out that not everyone is doing this to you.

In the past, you dressed up for your weight. If you had extra fat rolls and an overhang, you did your best to wear clothes to cover up your imperfections. I did the same thing. I would wear pants and judge my waist size for pants by buttoning my pants just below my belly button but on top of my overhang portion. I considered myself to not have a waistline. I dressed in sweatpants and rarely wore jeans. Most of my closet was stretch pants. My weight was constantly on my mind in the past. I can remember seeing other women in public thinking how they had no issues finding clothes to fit properly. Dressing up was a challenge because finding shirts to cover my bust was a problem as well. The extra fat around my upper back sections prevented me from wearing a bra that fit appropriately. I had to buy two sizes too big just to be able to latch both sides on the back. I once had a position at a local photography studio. I was so overweight that a button up shirt did not cover my body parts appropriately and I was forced to wear safety pins to hold the buttons in place on the front of my shirt. I got written up multiple times due to my pants not being business dress pants. I always wore black stretch pants. It was the only thing I had that would cover up my behind. I was so embarrassed some days at work with having to keep going to the dressing room to rearrange my clothing for work. Showing up for work with dress code violations is a strict indicator that most of the day you will be back and forth fixing yourself back up. I call this an "Epic Fail".

Appearing for the show to begin starts as soon as you leave home. From rearranging your bra, pants, and shirt as soon as you walk out of the door, all the way until you arrive at work. By the time I would arrive at work, I would be exhausted from the workout of getting ready for the day. Some days you dread appearing on stage at work and other public places because you already have in your mind negative thoughts of what others are going to say or think about you. The past experiences you have had play a major role into the way you view yourself now. If you were treated terrible overweight, it becomes a common normality for you and eventually you just accept it. Acceptance of being overweight is a great step in the right direction for uncovering who the real you is underneath all of that extra fat and skin. Finding yourself underneath all of the extra fat and skin can be a challenge for sure. Who you are on the outside does not determine who you are on the inside. You may have a heart of gold on the inside, but if you continue to see yourself and define yourself as the person from your past, you are holding yourself back.

You cannot move forward successfully if you are still living in the experiences of your past. I struggle with this so much. When I get down on myself, even now that I am thin, I find myself rewinding myself to the past words of others judgments about my weight. Getting beyond these feelings has caused me to look deeper inside of my own self instead of viewing who I am by my outer appearance. Taking myself away from the mirror and the scale has greatly changed my thinking. This wasn't a permanent disengagement, but simply a vacation from the opinions of the world and replacing them with the real opinions I have of myself. A "mental health" vacation is sometimes what you need. By taking myself away from the opinions of others, I have discovered how therapeutic it is to write and express myself in my book. Instead of going to a mental health counselor to have them give me medications for something I don't have, it has been more therapeutic for me to do what I am doing. It is more of a healing from the inside. When I got my inside thinking right, my outside followed in pursuit. You don't work on yourself for others. You work on yourself for you. When you uncover the real you, your stage is not the stage of others for you to perform on. The stage you create is the one you stand firm on in who you are. Be firm in who you become. As you journey through weight loss recovery, think of how far you have come when you think you want to revisit your past. There is nothing in your past for you except negativity and negative feelings associated with that negativity. Be strong and have faith in yourself. Recovering from the past mistake of others hurting you and messing with the feelings you have of yourself will only send you going back in the wrong direction. You want to keep moving forward to discovering who you are.

Now is the time for your Breakthrough! Do it for yourself!

Revealing Me - A Poem of Searching for Me

Revealing Me

In my reflection I see the same me,
Not who I am now
But the same old me.
Others notice the change in me
But I am blind to seeing everything
But the same old me.
People see me and say
"Look at you
You're melting away"
The inside of my heart wants to see
Everything they see of me
Everything I wish I could be.
Half of a year has gone by
And everyday all I do is try
Try to see the new me
The one all of you see.
My eyes are open
Im looking to find
The person Im going to be in my mind.
Losing lots of weight
Losing most of my hair
Sometimes I wonder if life is fair.
As time goes by
My eyes look up to the sky
And now I realize
And I know why
God has brought me to this place
In my life, but now I know why.
Melting away, shedding away
All the numbers on the scale
The shedding of my old life
And the coming of a new.
The time is here.
The time is now.
No time for fear.
No time to be a no show.
My life is at stake.
Time to change.
Time to get in shape.
Time for my heart
To be equal with my new shape.
The reflection I used to see
Is now me.
The person i am supposed to be
Have been
And always will be.
Time for love to fill my heart

And bring me closer
And not apart.
Closer to discovering me
Who i always have been
And who i am on my journey to be.

This is a poem I wrote about my changing views of myself. Who I see in the mirror is sometimes different than what others see. As my transformation continues, my personal views of myself will change too.

Breakthrough

Breakthrough

It's time to break through
Break through these chains,
The chains holding all this weight
The chains holding me back.

Breakthrough
Break through these chains,
These walls,
These pains.
These pains holding me back
And keeping me hostage
Keeping me from getting back on track.

Breakthrough
Break through these walls,
Oh, If they could talk
And say whats made me call
Call for a break through
From my downfall.

Breakthrough
Break through is coming
Coming like a train
Ready to shed the pain,
The tears,
The shame,
Shed all my fears.

Breakthrough
Break through these fears,
Shine like the sun,
Shedding more tears
To claim my victory is almost won.

Breakthrough
Break through has come
My victory has won.
The hurt and shame
From the weight I used to carry
Has broken through the chains,
Breaking through the chain
And releasing me from being held back
From the life I'm on my way to regain.

Breakthrough
Break through is here.
Broken through the chains,
The tears,

The pain,
The fears.
All are gone.
Victory is mine.
Breakthrough is here,
Shining like the sun,
My battle is won.

Breakthrough

Finding the Proper Care Afterwards

After surgery, you will need to spend some time finding the proper care afterwards. Your body will not be the same. Mine was so different after my surgery. I was no longer at a high risk of having another stroke, continuing high blood pressure medications, and no longer having seizures. Just because I did not have these issues anymore doesn't mean I quit going back to have regular checkups with my physicians. If anything, I stayed on top of my healthcare. I eventually got to discontinue all of my medications I was on before my surgery. I did keep my appointments I had previously scheduled.

As I came off my medications, my need for other types of physicians increased. I got a referral to a local chiropractor who helped to get my spine back in shape. He did some decompression therapy as well as worked with me on stomach tightening exercises. I learned how to do proper muscle toning and taking the right steps to tone my muscles that had been so out of shape for so long. I went to my chiropractor for 3 hours a week and received heat therapy on my back in ten minutes increments. This helped to waken up my muscles and get them ready for physical fitness. Running to the gym immediately after surgery is going to cause yourself overkill. You are setting yourself up for failure because the muscles you are working on and toning have been asleep for such a long time and getting the shock of their life. It's like they were being woken up from a deep sleep. I wore myself and my muscles out at the gym doing what I THOUGHT would help. Seeing a chiropractor is key to your spine getting straightened back out. My spine was leaned over and in so much pain from carrying around so much weight that it hurt when I sat down and when I stood up. As I continuously saw my chiropractor for six months, the pain was almost healed up and I could sit and stand up straight again. When I was overweight, my body would lean forward. Now I can sit straight up and cross my legs. Small accomplishments along your journey will keep you focused. Six months after surgery, I did become pregnant and had to discontinue my chiropractic care, but the lessons my chiropractor taught me will stay with me for a long time.

I did keep my family physician as well. I kept her for my after care because my surgeon could only help me with issues related to the surgery itself. My surgeon and my Primary care physician both stayed in contact when it was time for major decisions to be made regarding my health. It is a great idea as well to have everyone involved in your after care. The physicians who used to write you prescriptions for your medications should be followed up with every three months. As I have gained weight back due to my pregnancy right now, I have had to depend on my seizure physician to give me guidance. My seizures pretty well dissolved up until I got pregnant at six months post surgery. I have only gained around eighteen to twenty pounds and am right at the 5 and a half month mark in my pregnancy. My Obstetrician could not answer questions about taking care of myself and my unborn regarding medication during pregnancy, so once again I had to depend on my neurologist.

Many times throughout my recovery, I have had to go back to my primary care physician and my neurologist to get advice regarding the dispensing of medications during my pregnancy. When your body loses a massive amount of weight, it will go through so many changes in such a short time. My body needed time to heal. Just having someone there to call on was enough reassurance when I needed it. My hair started falling out at 3 months and I have had to take different types of supplements to help with my hair loss and have had to depend on my weight loss surgeons advice, but my primary care physicians prescription pad. There are many times you will discover there are issues within your new body that you need to see other kinds of physicians for and will need a referral from your primary care physician to be seen. This was my case with my bladder. From all of the weight I had carried for so long, my bladder would feel like it was falling. I had to be seen at a Urologist because it would not hold in urine for almost a month. My bladder would leak at times and I had to wear panty liners until the urologist put me on medications for two months. This was so aggravating and embarrassing. There will be times you will be embarrassed after surgery for things beyond your control. You just have to wear a smile and keep moving forward.

One of the key points in your recovery is finding the proper care after surgery. Whether it be a physician you have never seen before or seeing a chiropractor, you will definitely have to stay on top of your healthcare. Letting yourself go because you are dropping weight so fast will only lead to failure and cause you to become sick. Sick is not an option after surgery. The point of surgery is to get your body healthy again. Taking vitamins and supplements are going to be something you will have to do your entire life so you might as well get used to it being an everyday routine for you. Without vitamins and supplements, your body will get sick and you can cause your body to do things it normally would not do. Take care of yourself and your second chance in life.

Closet Full of Clothes

Now that the weight is falling off, you are struggling to find clothes that fit properly. The biggest struggle for me has been going into a store and running straight to the 2X and 3X sizes. I will grab all the beautiful ones I see and take my new haul to the dressing room to try everything on. After the first two shirts and pants, you try to do your best to not cry but your emotions will overwhelm you to the point where you see yourself in the mirror sobbing. You aren't sobbing tears of sadness, but tears of joy. The sadness you used to carry when clothes shopping is long gone. This sadness has been restored with joy. Tears of joy are good for your heart and soul as it is a reflection of your inner thoughts, feelings, and your heart. Your heart is displayed by your emotions. Many times I have stood in the dressing room sobbing tears of sadness because the beautiful clothes I had picked out, didn't even half fit my body. I would spend hours in stores searching for beautiful clothes in my size with no luck. I can remember passing stores in the mall or avoiding stores I know that did not carry my clothing sizes. I saw myself as ugly and shopping soothed my pit of despair inside of me.

The clothes in my closet when I was overweight consisted of sweatpants, elastic waistband pants, and capris. I had to constantly pull my pants up all day to cover up the overhang of my stomach. It was so embarrassing in public but I did what I had to do. I wore the same black pair of stretch pants to work for weeks and months at a time washing them daily because I had nothing else that fit me. I prayed daily for nobody to notice. Nobody ever said a word. I can remember times wearing my work shirt and having to stuff my fat rolls into those black stretch pants just to cover up the over hang I had at the time. I hated those pants because workout pants don't have pockets to put your personal items in. I am also one of those people who hides their phone in their bra because they don't have pockets in any of their pants. I no longer have this problem and look back and laugh about the things I had to do when I had nothing else to do with my phone. During the summer, I was so overweight, that I sweated profusely and ended up wearing tank tops and cotton capris that were really stretch pants. The winter months were easier to hide my overweight body. I could pile on layers without anyone knowing how much weight I was hiding underneath my clothes. My closet during the summer also consisted of maxi dresses. I can remember wearing them and having to wear a shrug over the arms because my upper body structure was so heavy and overweight that my arms had sagging skin hanging off my underarm area.

My stomach was so huge in front of me that it was a struggle to get the proper breast coverage. I would buy strapless bra after strapless bra but none of them would hold my weight of my breasts up where they needed to be. My breast size was 42DD. Currently, I am down to a C cup. You will go through a phase while losing weight where you will go down in bra sizes so fast that you have a different size every week. If you are like me, you have beautiful bras that are way too big now and you just can't stand to throw them away. I had a bra party and donated all of mine to the local women's shelter as well as many of my overweight clothes I could not consign or give away to anyone else. The women's shelter is a great resource to donate your lightly used bras to. Consider it gifting to other women in need. Don't donate your panties though. I had to trash my size 13 granny panties, and as I lose more weight, I am having to trash more of them. I don't spend a lot of money on undergarments right now due to such the drastic change in my overall health and weight.

The shoes in your closet are a discussion within themselves. What kind of shoes are in yours? I can tell you the two types of shoes I had when I was overweight. The first one was flip flops. Flip flops are basically the only shoe you can wear when your feet are so swollen. Flip flops were the staple in my closet. I couldn't even put on a single regular tennis shoe because the swelling in my feet caused them to hang over the sides of any pair of shoes I wore. My flip flops were worn down so much from all the excess weight I carried around that they had holes in their soles. I can remember the tongue coming out of them and being out in public having to buy another pair of flip flops because the ones I had on were so worn out. I wore my flip flops everywhere. When I was overweight, I hadn't owned a pair of regular tennis shoes in almost 7 years. I tried to wear flats and heels with no luck. Between the Plantar Fasciitis heel pain and the excess weight, I struggled to walk and struggled with daily tasks. I couldn't walk a treadmill nor walk my neighborhood block without having to sit down and take a rest.

You will experience so much within you as you transition into normal size clothing. The way you look at clothes will change as well as your mindset. When you go into a store, you will spend many hours in dressing rooms swapping out clothes to find the ones that fit you just right.

Surprise! You're Pregnant

Wow! Yes! Pregnancy can creep up on you and surprise you! It did for us! After nine years of not ovulating and having PCOS, my body just 'woke up". At three months post op (February 2016), my husband and myself took a trip to Hilton Head Island for our two year wedding anniversary. We had a great time on our second honeymoon, but we had a surprise when we got back home from our mini vacation. After getting sick and running a fever for two days, we went to the Emergency Room on Easter of 2016. I had no clue or even had a thought of pregnancy! We both thought I had gotten a stomach bug and was just sick from it. After three hours there, a doctor came in and told me my blood work showed I was pregnant. We were both in complete shock and started crying tears of joy! The five years we have been together, we have tried to have a baby, but my body just wouldn't cooperate or ovulate. There are times you are just in shock and just thanking God! We were so excited!

Little did we know, two months later our dreams were shattered. During spring break for our kids, we travelled around the country visiting different sights and destinations including the Rocky Mountains, Kentucky, and Texas. We had a great time, but on the first day of our trip, I started to have pains like I was having cramps. I did not think much of it at the time until I started to bleed a little. This bleeding turned into a flood in Kentucky. I called my doctor who thought I was just having regular implantation bleeding. I knew something else was going on. Throughout that week on the road, I continued to bleed clots, but was instructed it was just implantation or early trimester bleeding. When we got home at the end of that week, I went to my gynecologist who did my blood work and we received terrible news. My HCG levels were declining and I was miscarrying. This was in May 2016. We were just devastated and asking God why? Truly we will never know the answer to that question, but apparently God has a reason for everything. After my appointment with my gynecologist, I made an appointment to come back in a month (June 2016). I continued to bleed for almost 4 weeks. My doctor basically stated that I miscarried because my body could not support a healthy pregnancy with all of the changes I was still going through with my surgery being so recent.

We did come back for my follow up appointment for blood work. At the time, we did not know that God's answer to our prayers had come upon us so quickly again. We received a call the following day telling us that our blood work revealed we were pregnant AGAIN! We were so excited! Now our excitement turned into fear and worry. When you get pregnant right after a miscarry, you worry even more about what is going to happen with your pregnancy. We waited a long time going back and forth between my Obstetrician each week hoping for a heartbeat. The worry led to sleepless nights as well. Even with no heartbeat, our worry was escalated by continuous spotting and bleeding with trips to the Emergency Room to check on our baby. Finally at nine weeks, our doctor found a heartbeat. We just cried tears of happiness. Currently, I am at twenty weeks and we just found out we are having a girl after being told we were having a boy because of blood work results.

This pregnancy has been so different than with my nine year old daughter. I have gained very little weight. With my nine year old, I gained over 120 pounds and had gestational diabetes. I currently only get sick in the morning time compared to all day sickness with my nine year old. I don't crave a lot of food like my first pregnancy. My body needs proteins to keep me stomach intact, but my body rejects those foods and I throw them up. I have had to resort to light carbohydrates just to satisfy my body's needs for hunger. Eating these carbohydrates has caused me to have high sugars in my urine, high ketones, and early signs of diabetes. In my previous pregnancy, I had to do the glucose testing at my OB. With this pregnancy, I am exempt from the glucose test and having to just do a test for fasting.

The glucose test will cause me to go into "Dumping Syndrome". The rapid dumping of food into the body triggers the pancreas to release excessive amounts of insulin into the blood stream. The glucose drink is to determine high blood sugars in pregnancy and to diagnose gestational diabetes. The drink consists mostly of sugars and can cause people with weight loss surgeries to go into diabetic shock. To get exempt from this, I had to get my surgeon to send over a notice to my OB for my healthcare. I go for my "fasting" test in two weeks and hope it will help determine why my ketones stay so high. We are also thankful that we have no health issues with our baby. My blood work came back clear of any abnormalities.

Many people asked me why I was not using any birth control pills. After my stroke, my physicians would not prescribe me any medications due to the risk of stroke again. I am allergic to many contraceptives. I am married and we truly just didn't see pregnancy on our radar at this point. We are blessed to be having our baby and looking forward to my return back to my weight loss goals after she is born. When I found out I was pregnant this time, I had to cancel my skin removal surgery, which was scheduled in October 2016. I already had my insurance approved and my surgeon was already taking measurements when we found out we were pregnant. My surgery is rescheduled for next fall. I am excited to be able to get back on my protein eating track after the birth of our baby. So Yes! You can get pregnant quickly after surgery! Yes! There is a possibility of miscarry due to surgery complications! Taking care of yourself is vital to your health!

Where Do I Go From Here?

"Where do I go from here?"

This is probably the most asked question you will have after your surgery. I know it has been mine. Where do I go from here? What do I do with my life? Let me rephrase the question to "What do I do with my new life?" Where do I take myself on my next journey and how do I pick up where I feel my life left off before I gained the extra weight? Where does my heart go? Do I follow it? Do I step out and take that chance? Where do I go after "dumping my extra baggage?" Who am I?

Lots of questions and many answers out there but truly only you can find the answers to these questions. These answers lie within yourself. To find these answers you have to search within yourself. I can only answer these questions for me. I have had so much time to reflect over my life and how much God has truly blessed me. My heart will always feel pain and hurt from the way that others have been allowed to step into my heart to affect the way I feel about myself. I allowed my own self to judge myself based on others opinions. That is no longer my present, but my past. My present doesn't include others opinions of me anymore. When people look my way, I no longer try to read what they are feeling and thinking of me because I know that truly I am who I am. No excessive weight or others opinions of my body affect the way I view myself anymore. In my heart, I know who I am and what I am. I see a new life in my heart that just needed a revival. I needed to be revived from slowly killing myself from depression from the extra weight I used to carry. When a revival takes control in your heart, you are unstoppable.

I do not look back and try to pick up the pieces where I left off before I gained all of this weight because looking back isn't moving forward. There is nothing left for me in my past that my new life needs. I must look forward to the things I can do again. I am able to be on the soccer fields with my family. I am able to once again go swimming without feeling like my heart is going to stop. I get up early each morning and ready to go for the day. I have no signs of a stroke, heart attack, high blood pressure, or seizures. Most importantly I am "Mom" again. Many more things are to come for me.

One of my greatest feats this summer was to jump off the diving boards at our local swimming pool. I haven't jumped off a diving board in years, much less the high dive. For my daughter's ninth birthday party, I started on the low dive and I finally got up the nerve to jump off the high dive. My heart was pounding out of my chest for fear of sinking and not being able to come up. That past feeling of being scared back when I was overweight started to creep in on me. I immediately pushed it aside and thought of my accomplishments over the past 6 months and how far I have come. I decided that nothing can defeat me. I approached the end of the board and just jumped. The thrill set in as I hit the water and I came up in tears. Tears of joy took over in me as I came out of the water because I was finally able to do something I had always dreamed of doing but not been able to do because of my health situation. When you get that first accomplishment out of the way, you are unstoppable. Nothing can keep fear in you more than fear itself.

Throughout the past year since my surgery, I have saw my life change dramatically for the good. I no longer fear going into the grocery store alone cause I am worried about how others feel about me. To take control of your life and where you're future is going depends on you. What you do with the lessons you learn on your weight loss journey affect you and the others around you. Others are seeing you and how your life is changing. Many will accept your new changes and many will walk away. Let them walk away because sometimes you have to let go of everything and let God take care of things for you. My future from here has no plans except to live out my new life the best way I know how and let God take care of the rest.

Enjoy your journey and help others along the way! Get out there and make a change in the world. You have time to do the things you have missed out on!

Pictures of Me Now

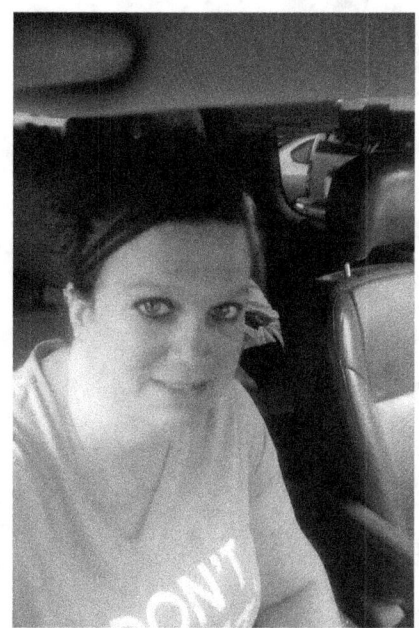

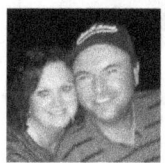

MY JOURNEY TO LOVING
MYSELF

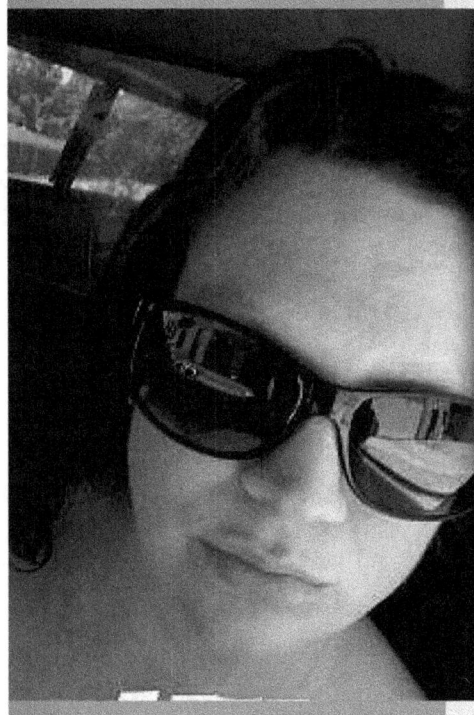

Gastric
Sleeve:
The
New
Me

LET YOUR FEAR BECOME
YOUR VICTORY

MINDY MITCHELL

www.ingramcontent.com/pod-product-compliance
Lightning Source LLC
Chambersburg PA
CBHW080442290526
45791CB00008BA/2580